HAIR & MAKE-UP

ACKNOWLEDGEMENTS

I would like to thank Catie Ziller for her ongoing support and for believing in me from start to finish with this project, and Anne Wilson, Jackie Frank and Matt Handbury for the opportunity to develop the concept. Special thanks to Debbie Pike for her endless enthusiasm, outstanding creativity and, most importantly, her great friendship. Thanks to David Parfitt for his innovative photography, brilliant eye and hours of hard work, and to Troy Word for his energy, creativity and ability to capture the spirit of this book on film. Special thanks also to Linda Hay for all her amazing make-up and to Tim Crespin for his great hairdos. To models Glenna, Melissa, Kim, Susan, Audrey and Carolyn for all your help and enthusiasm; to my editor, Lesley Levene, for making sense of this all and always being so calm; to my sister, Susie, for her endless support, drive and for keeping me sane – I couldn't have done this book without you; and to Stewart for the laughs that kept me going, to Brenda for her inspiration and to Brian for always being so level-headed, and to all my friends, especially Nicola, Nicky, Brendan and Sam and Michael, for being so understanding and supportive while I've been working on this book.

This edition published in the United States and Canada by Whitecap Books.
First published by Murdoch Books®, a division of Murdoch Magazines Pty Ltd, 45 Jones Street, Ultimo NSW 2007

Art director/designer: Debbie Pike. Still-life photographer: David Parfitt. Beauty photographer: Troy Word. Stylist: Jane Campsie.
Make-up: Linda Hay for Linda Hay Inc. Hair: Tim Crespin. Models: Glenna Neece, Kim Vos, Carolyn Park, Susan Carman, Melissa Keller, Audrey Quock.
Editor: Lesley Levene.
CEO & Publisher: Anne Wilson. Associate Publisher/Publishing Director: Catie Ziller. International Sales Director: Mark Newman.

A catalogue record for this book is available from the National Library of Australia
ISBN 0 86411 805 8.
©Text Jane Campsie 1998. ©Design and photography Murdoch Books® 1998. Printed by Toppan Printing (S) Pte Ltd, Singapore. First printed 1998. PRINTED IN SINGAPORE.
Distributed in Canada by Whitecap Books (Vancouver) Ltd, 351 Lynn Avenue, North Vancouver, BC, V7J 2C4
Telephone (604) 980 9852 Facsimile (604) 980 8197 or Whitecap Books (Ontario) Ltd, 47 Coldwater Road, North York, ON, M3B 1Y8
Telephone (416) 444 3442 Facsimile (416) 444 6630
Distributed in the USA by Graphic Arts Centre Publishing, PO Box 10306, Portland, OR, USA, 97296-0306
Telephone (503) 226 2402 Facsimile (503) 294 9900

HAIR & MAKE-UP

JANE CAMPSIE

Still-life photography: David Parfitt   Beauty photography: Troy Word

WHITECAP
BOOKS

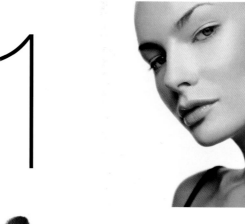
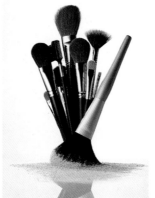
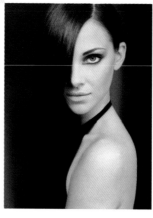
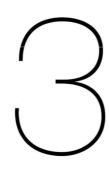
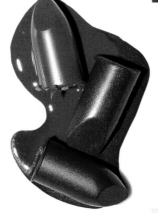
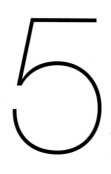
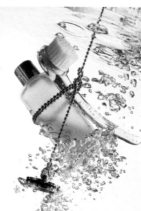

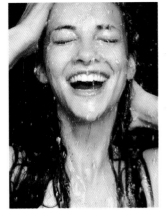

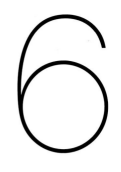
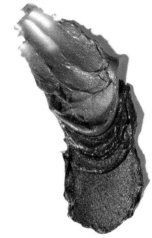

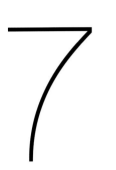
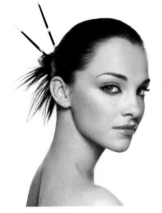

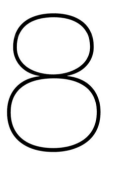
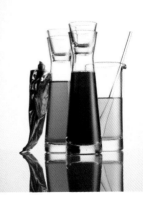

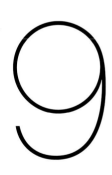
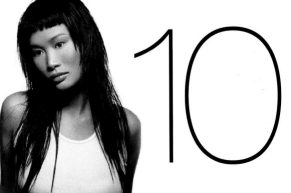

PHILOSOPHY

HAIR & MAKE-UP–This definitive guide to looking good offers a realistic approach to modern beauty to boost your self-esteem and confidence. It is not about following the latest make-up trends, wearing the colour of the moment or sporting the most fashionable hairstyle, it is about adapting different looks to suit you, in order to accentuate your best features to bring out your natural beauty. So whether you have never really explored the potential of experimenting with different hairstyles and make-up, or if you are stuck in a beauty rut or simply wanting a change, use this book to your advantage. There are no strict rules and regulations as to what you can and can't do when it comes to hair and make-up. The secret is to find what suits you and your lifestyle. In keeping with the pressures of modern living, it is essential to find ways to maintain hair upkeep and perfect your make-up at high speed, without cutting back on the results, all the time aiming to make looking good a simple task. I hope that you will find this book easy to follow and will reap the benefits, improving the way you look and feel and, most importantly, enjoying yourself in the process.

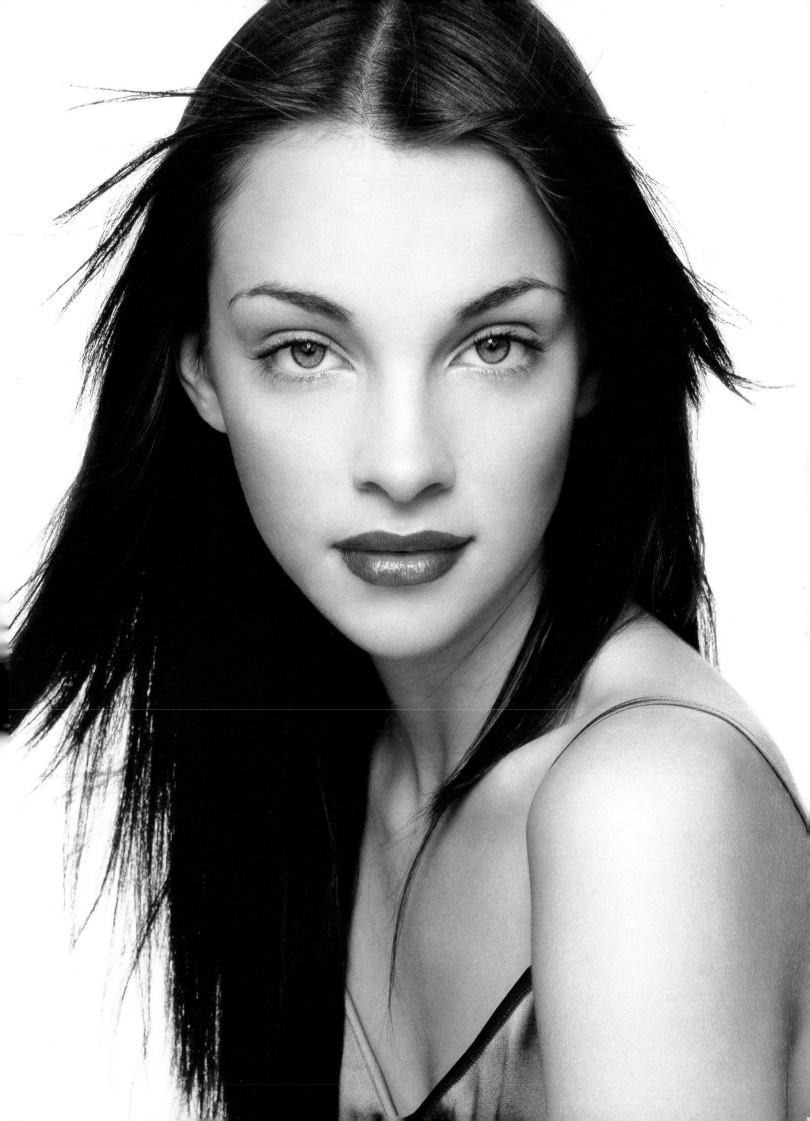

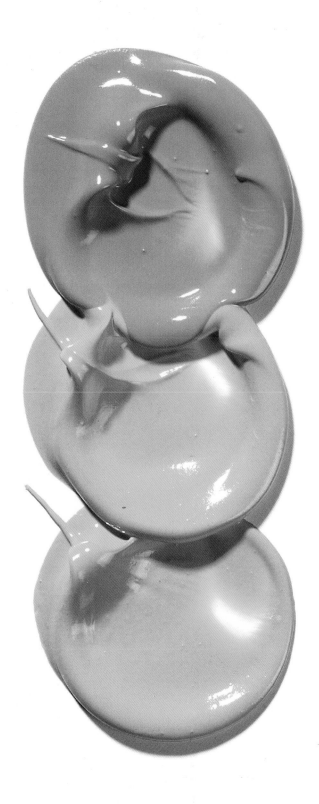

bare essentials

1

Make-up should be used to help you look good and feel better. Find your own basic make-up essentials to create a radiant-looking complexion and then experiment with different colours, textures and cosmetic items to accentuate your features and enhance your face. Improving your appearance will boost your confidence and self-esteem.

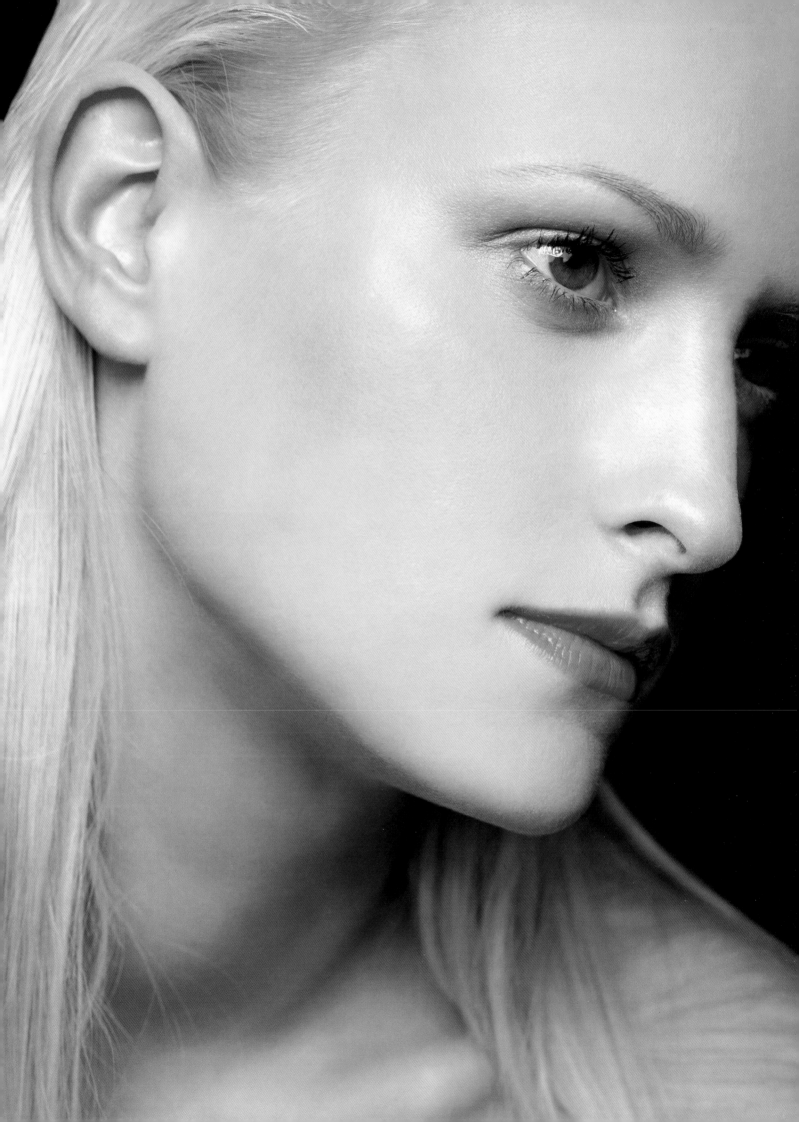

MAKE-UP
ESSENTIALS

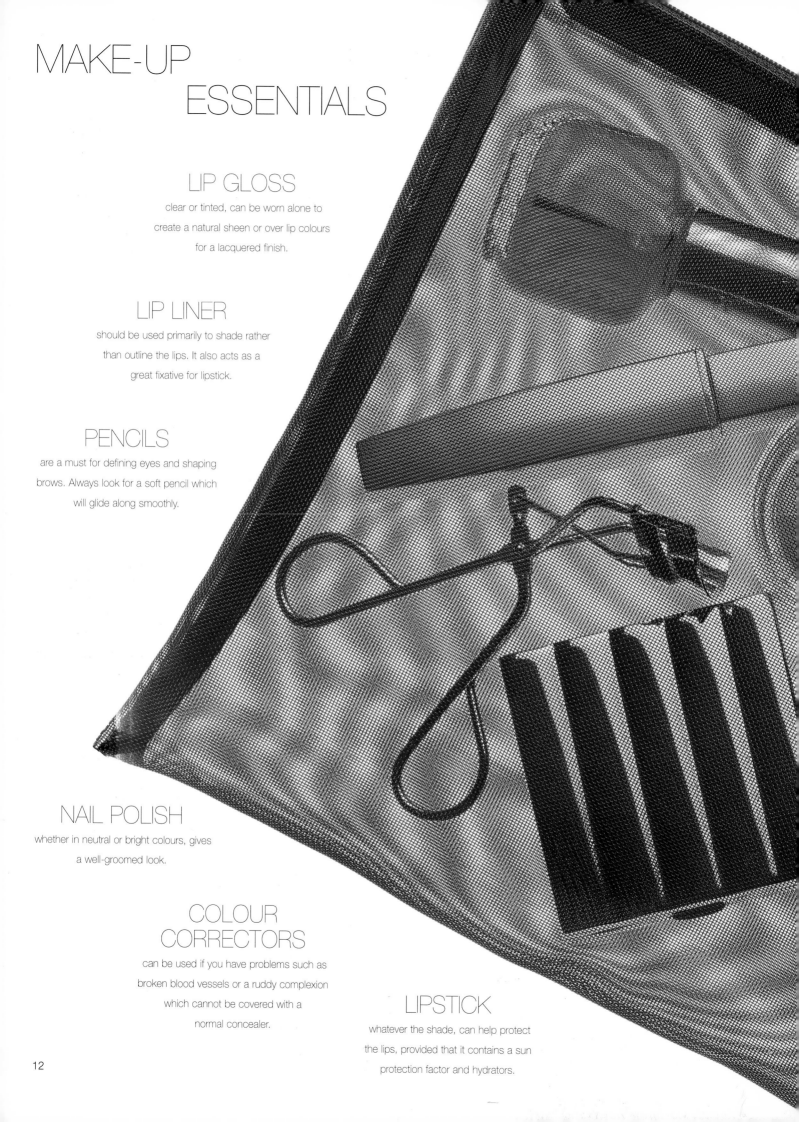

LIP GLOSS

clear or tinted, can be worn alone to
create a natural sheen or over lip colours
for a lacquered finish.

LIP LINER

should be used primarily to shade rather
than outline the lips. It also acts as a
great fixative for lipstick.

PENCILS

are a must for defining eyes and shaping
brows. Always look for a soft pencil which
will glide along smoothly.

NAIL POLISH

whether in neutral or bright colours, gives
a well-groomed look.

COLOUR
CORRECTORS

can be used if you have problems such as
broken blood vessels or a ruddy complexion
which cannot be covered with a
normal concealer.

LIPSTICK

whatever the shade, can help protect
the lips, provided that it contains a sun
protection factor and hydrators.

CONCEALER

in a retractable stick will give better coverage and last longer than creamy formulations. Look for a shade with a yellow undertone to suit your skin tone.

LOOSE POWDER

must be super-fine to ensure it creates a 'barely there' finish and looks as natural as possible once applied.

PRESSED POWDER

is ideal for retouches when you're on the move and is easy to apply, so it goes just where it's needed.

FOUNDATION

is essential to smooth the skin and disguise imperfections. Dry skin needs a creamy formulation and oily skin will benefit from an oil-free compact or liquid foundation. For superior coverage, choose a liquid or stick foundation.

TINTED MOISTURIZER

is great if your skin requires minimal coverage and you find foundation too heavy. In the summer choose one with a sun protection factor.

MASCARA

accentuates the lashes, helping to frame the eyes. For the best results, two fine coats are better than one single, heavy-handed application.

LIQUID EYELINER

is essential for transforming daytime make-up into a glamorous evening look, but it does require precision application.

EYESHADOW

in striking, slightly shimmering tones, applied with a light hand, can give the face an air of luminosity.

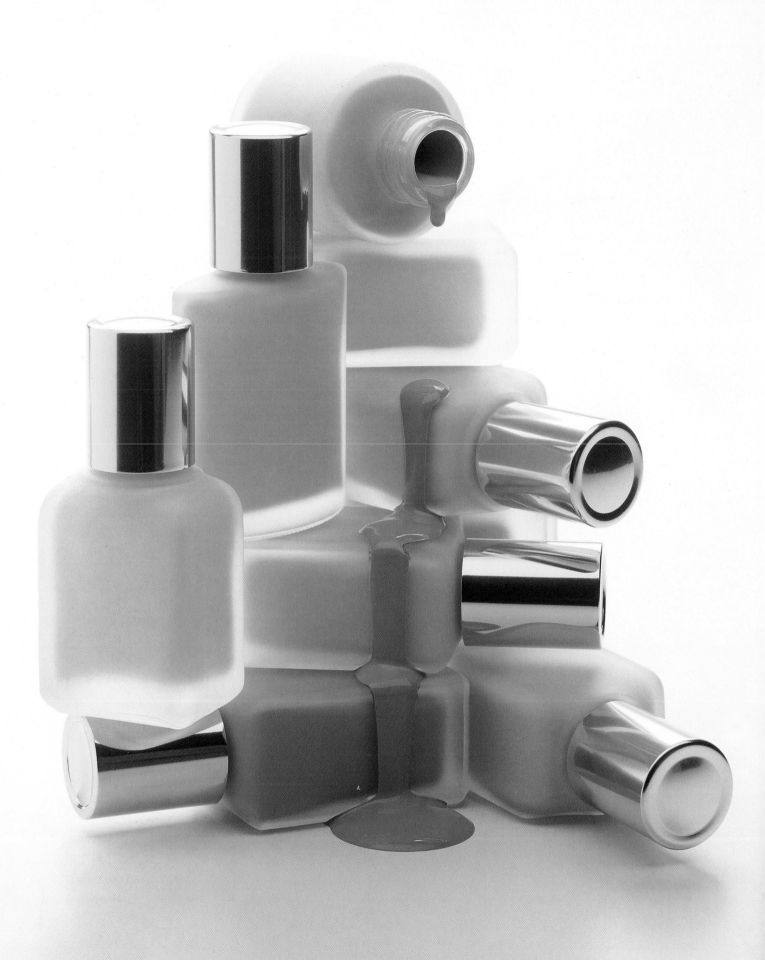

BASE WORK

FOUNDATION Applied properly, foundation can make any complexion seem healthy and flawless. The aim is to leave the skin looking as natural and unmade-up as possible. Before you start, think hard about your complexion, as you may not need to apply base over the entire face. When choosing a foundation, take into consideration your skin type, the amount of coverage you require and the kind of finish you are after. And remember, foundation is one of those products you wear every day, so making the right investment at the beginning will pay off.

FORMULATIONS Different foundations will provide different types of coverage. Stick formulas can be applied with the fingertips or a sponge, giving sheer to medium coverage. For the best results, smooth on in fine layers, gradually building up. It is much easier to add make-up than try to remove it after application. Compact foundations combine face powder and foundation in one. They are usually creamy formulations which dry to a matt finish and are available in oil-free versions. They can be applied wet, with a damp make-up sponge, to achieve greater coverage, or with a dry sponge for a more natural-looking finish. Compact foundations are a great option if you're pushed for time as they can create a base at high speed. Liquid foundations give good coverage and they come in different finishes. Tinted moisturizers and aerated mousse formulations give minimal coverage, making them ideal for younger skins.

SKIN TYPES If you have sensitive skin, look for formulations which do not contain potential irritants such as fragrance, chemical sunscreens and alpha hydroxy acids. Mature, dry skins will benefit from rich, creamy foundations which contain emollients to boost the skin's moisture content and antioxidants to protect from environmental damage. Oily, problem skins will benefit from oil-free formulations which are enriched with oil absorbers to keep unsightly shine at bay. Normal skins can wear any sort of foundation. In hot, humid weather, every skin type will benefit from an oil-free foundation.

SHOPPING FOR FOUNDATION To find the perfect foundation for your particular colouring, apply three suitable shades in strips across the cheek and jawbone. You are looking for the one that literally disappears into the skin. Your foundation should blend with the skin tone of the neck and not the face, as this is where it has to work down to. If you can't find the correct colour, custom-blended foundations are available. When you try a new shade, check it in natural light. You should always aim to apply your make-up in daylight, so if this is not going to be possible invest in a natural daylight bulb (these can be found in lighting stores and some professional make-up outlets). When trying a new foundation, always wait fifteen minutes before reaching a decision as the oil on your skin and the air can conspire to darken the shade you have chosen.

FOUNDATION ESSENTIALS When looking for a new foundation, bear in mind that it should contain a sun protection factor of at least 15 for daily use. This should then be increased in summer, as the sun is responsible for 90 per cent of premature ageing. Antioxidants will also help protect the skin from visible signs of ageing, and light-reflecting pigments will give a flattering finish, taking attention away from any dark circles and sallow-looking areas, while adding instant luminosity.

EXPERT ADVICE To apply foundation, start from the centre of the face, dotting on to the cheeks and forehead and blending outwards, first making sure your fingertips or make-up sponges are spotlessly clean. Gently blot the skin with a tissue to remove any excess product or surface oil. Never drag the skin if you are using your fingertips to apply cosmetics. Smooth foundation over the lips and eyelids to act as a base for lip and eye products. If you're not very good at blending foundation, try applying it with a make-up sponge. After smoothing on, moisten the fingertips and then work over the neckline to remove any signs of haphazard application.

UNDER COVER

CONCEALER If you do not have a flawless complexion, concealer will be one of the most valuable cosmetics in your quest for beauty perfection. It can be used to disguise broken capillaries, dark circles, pimples and blemishes, and to even out skin tone. For the best all-round coverage, opt for a stick concealer (creamy and liquid concealers can be quite oily and have a tendency to slide on and glide off, creasing on the face, whereas stick formulas will stay put). The only drawback with them is that they can be more difficult to blend. To overcome this, work the stick up and down the back of your hand. The product will warm up, making it more pliable and so easier to use. Apply it with the fingertips so that it literally melts into the skin. Those with dry skin will need a concealer with emollients to counteract dryness, while those with oily, problem skins will need a concealer which stays put, is oil-free and contains antibacterial ingredients to help treat blemishes and spots.

SHADE SELECTION To counteract blueness and dark circles under the eyes, go for a concealer with a yellow undertone that is one to two shades lighter than the colour of the skin itself. If concealer is being used to mask pimples, to even out skin tone or to tone down broken capillaries, ensure that the shade you choose has a yellow undertone (pinkish shades will only accentuate redness) and is a good match for the natural colour of your skin. Make-up artists advise testing concealer shades on the inside of the forearm.

APPLICATION Always apply your concealer on top of foundation and before you add powder. If you try to do things the other way round, you might wipe the concealer off when applying your foundation. To disguise under-eye darkness, gently pat concealer under the eyes using the index finger. Exert only gentle pressure and blend outwards, taking care not to drag the skin. To conceal bags under the eyes, put concealer on the shadow beneath the bag, not on the bag itself, otherwise you'll end up highlighting rather than hiding the problem. To cover up broken capillaries or uneven skin tone, you can either massage concealer into the skin or paint it on with a brush and blend with the fingertips. To touch out any blemishes or unsightly-looking spots, paint on concealer with a brush. Remember to start at the centre of the imperfection and feather outwards.

PROBLEM SOLVERS If your concealer dries and cakes in fine lines and wrinkles around the eyes, try using an eye cream under the concealer; make sure you use only a small amount of concealer and opt for one with a matt finish to create the illusion of smooth skin. To prevent the concealer highlighting a problem you're trying to hide, apply a light moisturizer as an undercoat. Allow it to soak in and then dab away any excess with a tissue. This will make the skin soft and more even to work on. For extra staying power, once you have applied concealer, especially over pimples, set with a light dusting of sheer powder. If concealed areas dry out and start to flake throughout the day, gently pat on a small amount of moisturizer.

COVERING SCARS Scars or birthmarks can be disguised using heavy-duty concealers. As additional coverage is required, it's best to buy a preparation from a specialist make-up store, not a general cosmetic counter. Concealers designed for television will give great coverage and are available in water-resistant and waterproof formulations to ensure they stay put in a range of different circumstances.

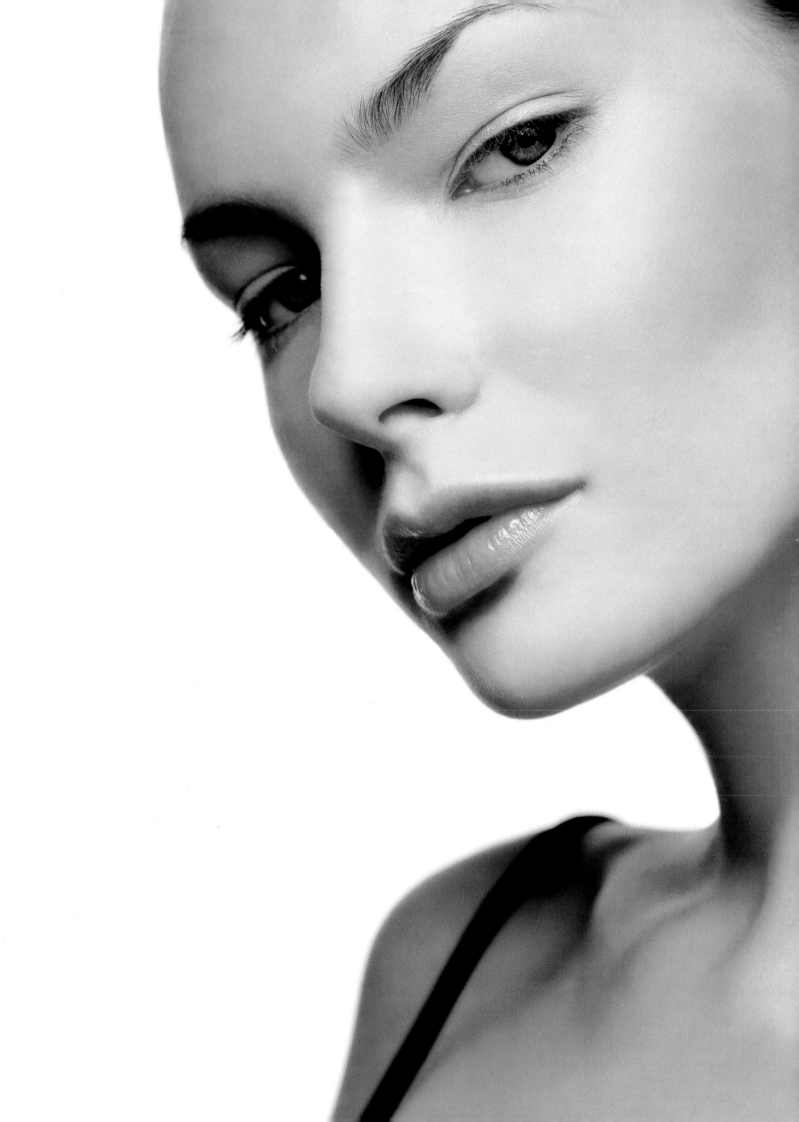

POWDER
FINISH

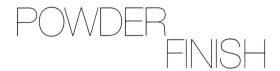

POWDER Face powder can be one skin type's ally and another's arch enemy. Oily skins will benefit from face powder which contains special oil-absorbing ingredients to give the skin a matt finish and mop up unsightly oil secretions. After several hours' wear, if the skin starts to look shiny, blot it with a clean tissue to absorb excess surface oil and then touch up with face powder. If you have dry skin, then go lightly with the powder; otherwise you will only accentuate the dryness. If you are using a foundation which aims to create a dewy-looking finish, avoid using any powder at all.

FORMULATIONS Decisions as to loose or pressed powder are a matter of personal preference. Loose powder is ideal to use when you're at home but is impractical to carry around, while pressed powder is great for retouches when you're on the move and is much easier to control. If you have a tendency to be heavy-handed when applying make-up generally, steer clear of loose powder.

COLOUR CHOICE Opt for a yellow-toned powder instead of a translucent shade to warm the skin. Translucent powders are not, as most people imagine, invisible; they can zap the natural colour of the skin and make complexions look pasty. To determine if a powder is good quality, test it on the back of your hand; it should feel silky and smooth and very light. If it looks chalky and heavy, this means it has not been finely milled – which will show up on the face.

APPLICATION Leave your foundation to settle for a couple of minutes before dusting on powder. There is no need to apply powder all over the face. Aim to keep your complexion looking as fresh and dewy as possible. Use powder mainly on areas of the face that are prone to shine, such as the chin, nose and forehead. For the best results when applying face powder, dust on with a brush in small swirling motions over the face and then sweep the brush downwards. This will remove any excess powder that has collected around the eyebrows or under superfluous facial hair and will ensure that these hairs lie flat on the face. If you want to use loose powder but are not confident about your ability to control the brush, try dusting the powder into the palms of your hands, then rubbing your hands together gently and pressing them over your face. Finally run a large brush over your face to remove any excess powder.

EXPERT ADVICE Take a tip from the make-up artists: they advise blowing gently on a loaded brush before applying powder, to remove any excess. Always remember that your make-up will take a few minutes to settle into the skin after application, but if you find that your complexion looks unnatural and artificial, spray with a fine mist of water or facial toner. It is worth investing in a small natural sea sponge to use to set your make-up. After applying your foundation and powder press the damp sponge lightly into your complexion. This will make your base look fresh and dewy, instead of powdery and lifeless.

BRONZING POWDER To give the complexion a radiant glow, you can always use bronzing powder instead of face powder. Look for a bronzer which is one or two shades darker than your skin tone – but avoid shades which are too dark, as they will look very unnatural and false. For the best results, dust bronzing powder on to the cheeks, tip of the chin, nose and forehead, and finish off by sweeping over the entire face. Bronzers laced with flecks of shimmer can add luminosity to the complexion, but if you have older skin choose a matt version for a more flattering finish.

EYE COLOUR

EYESHADOW This should always glide on smoothly, and can be used to subtly change or enhance the shape of the eyes, to add simple definition or to make a strong impact, depending on your choice of colour. It is also useful to disguise the blueness many of us have on the skin on our eyelids.

CREAM VS POWDER Whether you wear cream or powder formulations of eyeshadow is down to personal preference. Cream-to-powder eyeshadows are easy to apply, as they can be literally swept over the eyelid in one stroke, but they have the disadvantage of gliding off again within hours of application or of creasing in the eyelid. To improve the staying power of cream eyeshadow, try setting it with a light dusting of translucent powder. While powder eyeshadows do tend to stay put, they require greater precision in application. Older skins will benefit from the use of powder eyeshadows.

COLOUR CHOICE When you select colours, remember that dark ones deepen or hollow features, while light ones will make the eyes stand out. Choose bright colours carefully. They can look great but they draw attention instantly to the eyes and run the risk of looking unnatural, unless the face is balanced with other suitable make-up products. Don't be put off by eyeshadow colours before you have tried them, as most will appear more intense in the palettes than they actually are. Experiment with bright shades, but use them as a wash over the eyelids to add a subtle hint of colour. You don't need to wear colours that match the colour of your iris, but it's a good idea to select shades which will accentuate your natural colouring. For those with blue eyes, try liner in brown or navy and avoid wearing blue eyeshadow. Green eyes stand out when shaded with khaki and brown shades with yellow undertones. Very dark brown eyes can wear almost any colour but look especially striking with browns, charcoal and mahogany. Finally, grey/green eyes are enhanced by charcoal and black.

OPTICAL ILLUSION If you wear glasses, take into consideration the type of lenses you have when you are selecting make-up. If you are short-sighted, corrective lenses will magnify your eyes, so unless you have naturally small eyes wear muted or natural shades of eyeshadow. If you are long-sighted, your lenses will make your eyes appear smaller, so use eyeshadow to strengthen them. Dust eyeshadow along the socket line and outer corners of the eyes, but do not shade the eyelid heavily. Avoid wearing eyeliner on the upper lash line and steer clear of dark eyeshadow, as this will make the eyes appear smaller than they are. Also, frames will cast a shadow on the face, so disguise any darkness with a concealer one shade lighter than your foundation.

EXPERT ADVICE Make-up artists recommend that, when you are wearing eyeshadow, you should pile on extra loose powder under the eyes to catch any stray particles of eyeshadow. After shading the eyes, this can be removed by dusting off with a large make-up brush. After application, if you feel your choice of eyeshadow is too intense, tone the colour down by dusting with face powder or gently wipe a foundation sponge over the eyelid to make the overall effect more subtle. To ensure that your eyeshadow is long-lasting and crease-proof, make-up artists advise application with a damp make-up brush. As the eyeshadow is blended into the skin, it will dry. Also, because the product will cling to the wet brush, stray particles of powder will not collect on the cheeks.

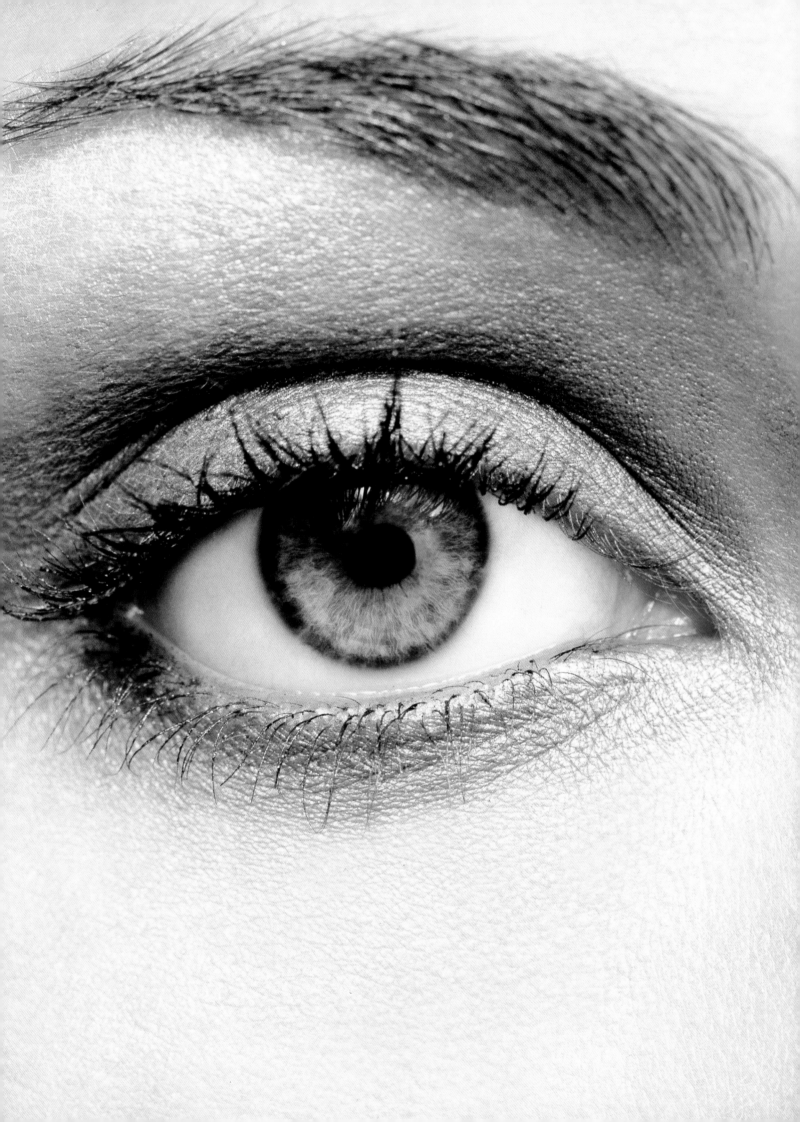

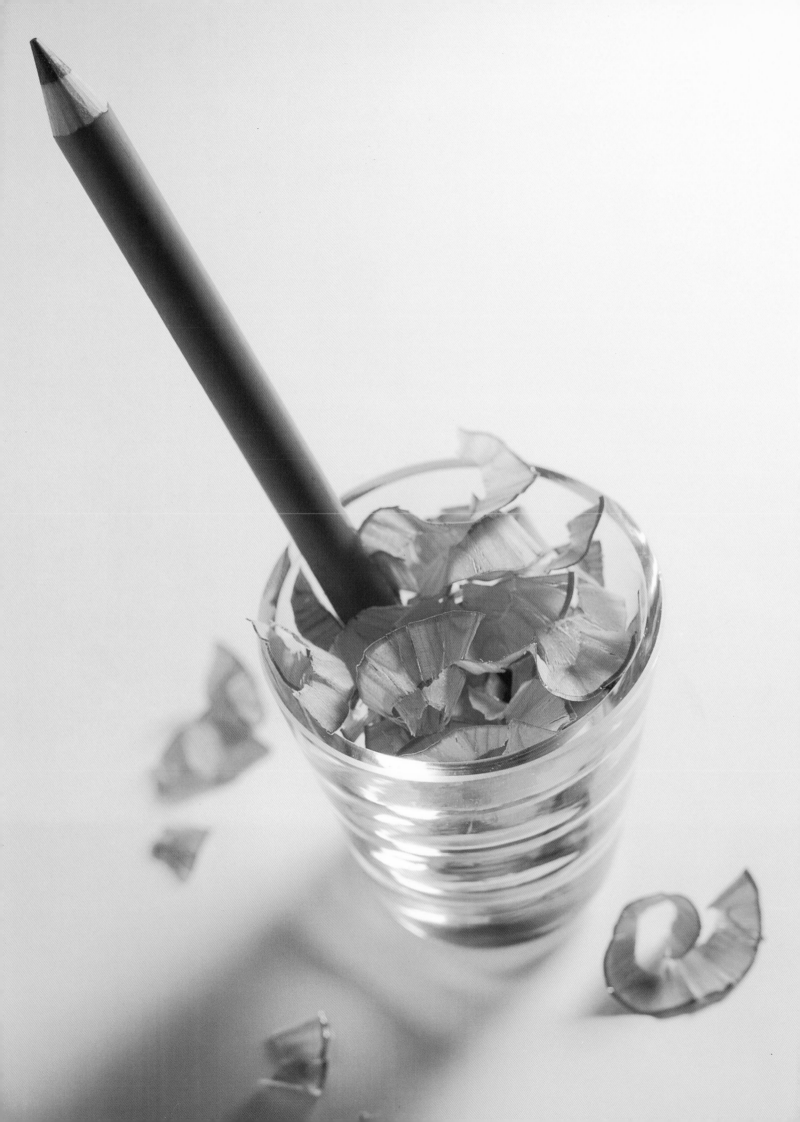

EYE DEFINITION

PENCILS Whether they are being used to shade or define the eyes, lips or brows, pencils should glide on smoothly, without dragging the skin. If they seem to be too soft and crumbly, place them in the freezer for a few minutes to harden before applying. If they are too hard and pull at the skin, soften the point first by gently running it over the back of the hand.

EYELINER Application requires a steady hand. If you find it difficult to apply liner with precision, try drawing it on using small feathered stokes and then blend with a fine-tipped brush or the point of a cotton bud. To make things easier, put a mirror on a flat surface and then work looking down into it. As an alternative to the visible pencil line on the eyes, try a join-the-dots approach. Dot pencil between the lashes and then run over the dots with a fine-tipped brush. If you do not have an eye pencil to hand, use a damp fine-tipped brush and paint on eyeshadow in a thin line. If you have naturally pale lashes but cannot reach the roots with a mascara wand, use liquid eyeliner, dabbing it on to cover them. It's worth investing in a white eyeliner: it could save the day on many occasions. If you're tired and your eyes don't look particularly sparkly, run a white pencil along the inner rim of the lower lash line. You will instantly look more awake and the whites of your eyes will appear brighter. It can also make small eyes appear larger. Never lend eye pencils to other people, as this is one of the quickest ways to spread germs. If you have an eye infection, replace eye pencils and mascaras to avoid reinfecting the eyes. Sharpen pencils regularly to ensure that the points are clean.

BROW PENCILS These can be used to fill sparse brows and enhance the overall shape. Take a sharpened pencil in the shade closest to the natural colour of your eyebrows and fill any open spaces using short irregular strokes to simulate real hair. When defining the brows, avoid drawing on one strong line as this will look false. Work over the brows in small feathered strokes. If the definition is too strong, soften it by dusting with translucent powder or roll a cotton bud over the brows.

MASCARAS As mascaras are now loaded with proteins and waxes to condition the lashes and come in problem-solving formulations, look for one that suits your needs. Thin, sparse-looking lashes will benefit from lash-building formulations that contain special ingredients to add volume and thickness. If you wear contact lenses, do not use lash-building mascaras, as the fibres within them can get trapped between eye and lens, causing irritation. Short lashes should be coated with mascaras containing plastic polymers which cling just to the tips of the lashes to create the illusion of extra length. Sporty and outdoor types should opt for a waterproof or water-resistant mascara (the former will withstand a dip in the pool, while the latter holds up only to tears or perspiration). These types of mascaras are extremely effective but can be drying on the lashes and have no ability to add volume or thickness to the lashes.

WONDER WANDS However refined the formula, the shape of the mascara wand plays a significant role in lash definition. For example, crescent-shaped wands will help curve the lashes up; fat wands with lots of bristles will help thicken the lashes by coating each one individually; bristleless wands (they look like the tip of a metal screw) will allow you to paint lashes right to the roots; and double-tapered brushes (they have small bristles at either end that get longer towards the middle of the wand) will help define very thin and sparse lashes.

EXPERT ADVICE With modern mascaras there is no need to pump the wand in and out of its container before applying. This can actually cause overload and result in clogged lashes. You need only enough product on the wand to coat the lashes, so any excess should be wiped off with a tissue. Roll the wand through the lashes to help curl-definition. Always work on the upper lashes from underneath to avoid overloading and keep mascara on the lower lashes to a minimum, especially if you are looking tired or have a tendency to rub your eyes a lot.

LIP FIX

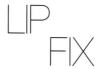

LIPSTICK This is one of the easiest and quickest ways to transform your appearance. You don't need to co-ordinate your lip colour with your nail polish or wardrobe, but you may want to take into consideration what you are wearing. It is essential to ensure that your lip colour blends with the rest of your make-up look and also complements your skin tone. Those with olive complexions should opt for colours with warm undertones to brighten the skin, such as light brown, raisin or brown reds, like blackberry and wine. Those with fair complexions need lip colours with warm peach or pink undertones, while those with pale complexions can wear almost any colour, using dramatic shades to make a strong beauty statement. Dark complexions look best with deep reds with dark blue or purple undertones or deep browns with purple, blue or wine undertones.

FINDING THE FORMULATION To test-run a

new shade, don't try it on the back of your hand. Instead, dab it on to your fingertip, where the colour of the skin is closest to that of your lips. This can also be held near your mouth, to see if the colour suits you. Once you have found the correct shade, you need to consider the effect you are after. Glossy finishes give sheer coverage but need to be reapplied frequently. Matt finishes give great coverage but have a tendency to be drying on the lips and can look very flat; to overcome this, look for demi-matt finishes, which dry to a more flattering finish. Creamy finishes create opaque coverage with a hint of shine and come enriched with conditioners, making them a suitable choice if your lips are prone to dryness. Sheer lipsticks give the lips a subtle wash of colour, similar to lip gloss, but are longer-lasting. They are ideal as lightweight options to wear during the summer. Lip gloss has a tendency to glide on and slide off within hours of application. To help it stay put, prime the lips with a lip pencil in the shade closest to the natural colour of the lips. Then apply gloss to the centre of the top and bottom lip and purse the lips together. This creates the illusion of all-over shine without the problem of disappearing gloss.

SHAPING UP If you apply lipstick without a brush, after a while it will acquire a shape. Experts have linked these shapes with personality types. If your lipstick has worn flat, this is an indication that you're a relaxed, sporty person who loves the outdoor life. If the tip is rounded, this shows that you're gentle and romantic. If it's worn to a strong, slanted edge, this means that you are articulate and well balanced. And if it's shaped like the top of a whistle (curved in at the sides, going up to a central tip), this means you're outgoing, with a dominating personality.

EXPERT ADVICE If you want to wear a dark lipstick

but doubt your application skills, use your fingertip and dab it on so the pigment stains the skin, then coat with lip gloss. To avoid leaving lipstick marks on glasses and cups, discreetly lick the rim before drinking. If lipstick always ends up on your teeth, place your middle finger in your mouth, pout and withdraw the finger. If you are pushed for time, avoid wearing dark or bright lipsticks as they need precision application and use gloss or a neutral-toned lipstick instead. If your lipstick has a tendency to bleed or feather into fine lines around the mouth, use a lip liner to shade the entire lip area before applying lipstick; also, wearing a lipstick that dries to a matt finish should help. Avoid wearing lipsticks with a frosted finish as you get older, since these will only highlight any lines around the mouth.

LIP PENCILS Do not use just to outline the lips – this looks very dated and you could be left with a unsightly line when your lipstick wears off – but to define and shade the entire lip area. This acts as a fixative for lipstick and ensures that your lip colour will fade evenly. For a natural look, apply in a series of small feathered strokes around the outer edges of the lips, then blend with the fingertips and shade over the lips with the liner. If your lips are dry, making the liner hard to manoeuvre, coat them with lip balm first and blot with a tissue before applying lipliner. You do not need to buy different-coloured lip liners to match different lipstick shades. Rather, choose one similar to your natural lip colour and use this to shade and define the lips.

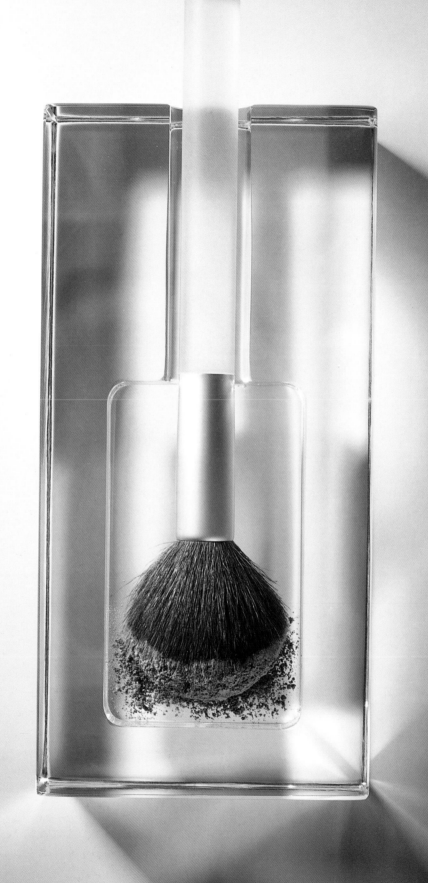

CHEEK COLOUR

BLUSHER If you haven't got razor-sharp cheekbones, don't worry: with the correct blusher you can achieve anything. Whether you wear a powder or a cream blusher, the secret is to create an effect which looks completely natural – unless, of course, you are going for the latest fashion look. With any cosmetic item, the choice between cream and powder formulations is a matter of personal preference. Cream or gel blushers literally melt into the skin and are easy to apply, while powder formulations can be dusted on at high speed. Make-up artists advise that you should team your choice of blusher with your foundation formulation: so, if you are wearing a creamy make-up base, go for cream blusher, and if your foundation dries to a powdered finish, dust on powder blusher.

SHADE SELECTION To find your most flattering shade of blusher, pinch your cheeks, study the shade and try to match it. For a natural-looking finish, opt for a shade of blusher that is one or two shades darker than your skin tone. If you go darker than this it will look unnatural. There is no need to invest in lots of different shades of blusher; you can buy one colour (such as a warm beige or soft brown) that will work with all make-up looks.

APPLICATION Always apply your blusher after the rest of your make-up. Then you can add the right amount to balance your overall look. A quick and foolproof way is to smile when you brush on colour to the cheek apples – that is, where you blush naturally. Use small circular motions to create a rosy-cheeked effect. Avoid enhancing the cheek apples if you have a particularly round face, as this will only accentuate the shape. To softly sculpt the cheekbones, again apply blusher in small circular motions, this time working down the cheekbone. This will prevent any unsightly stripes of colour occurring. To give the skin on the cheeks a smooth, poreless finish, stroke blusher downwards; if you go upwards, you run the risk of pushing pigment up and into your pores, thus highlighting any open ones. Always start applying colour at the top of the cheeks and work down. This way, the colour will gradually fade and you'll be left with the right amount of blusher in the right places.

EXPERT ADVICE Add blusher as the finishing touch to your make-up. The shade you wear does not have to match your lip and eye colour but it should be from the same colour family; otherwise it might disrupt the balance of the face. For example, wearing an orange blusher with red lipstick is not flattering, unless you want to make a statement. A darker than usual shade of face powder can be used in place of blusher. Face powders intended for black and Latina women are great choices as blushers for pale and medium-toned skin.

BLUSH MISHAPS If, having applied your blusher, you find it looks too dark to harmonize with your make-up, either buff it away with a velour powder puff and translucent powder or press a damp cosmetic sponge into the skin to lift off the colour. To ensure the problem does not arise in the first place, apply cheek colour lightly, remembering that it is better to build up colour gradually than go for one heavy-handed application.

CUSTOM BLENDING

BLUSHING FACES

If your summer blusher does not suit your paler winter face, dip the loaded blusher brush into translucent powder before dusting on. Create your own blusher by mixing a small amount of lipstick with face cream on the back of your hand and then dab on to the cheeks. Alternatively, dot a creamy lipstick on to the cheeks and gently blend into the skin.

IN THE MIX

You can mix existing products to create new colours and textures. To combine different lipsticks, either mix on the back of the hand using a lip brush or chop up the colours, place in a small dish and heat gently in the microwave for a couple of seconds, or until the lipsticks turn into a liquid. Pour into a palette and leave to set, before painting on with a brush.

POWDER PLAY

To blend loose face, eye or cheek powder, simply place in a bowl and mix together throroughly using a spatula. For a foolproof way to blend them, place in an air-tight container with a lid and shake vigorously. Pressed powders are best mixed on the back of the hand, using your fingertips or a make-up brush; or crush them together with a palette knife.

PERFECT SHADE

Black skin does not always have an even tone all over, so it can be difficult to find one single shade of foundation. Make-up artists recommend investing in three shades which are close to your natural skin tone and then mixing and matching these until you create the perfect colour combination to suit the different tones on your face.

mix cosmetics to create new colours and textures

SHEER TINTS
If your make-up bag is full of brightly coloured or extremely dark lip shades which you never wear, customize them with Vaseline. Prime the lips with Vaseline and then paint on lip colour with a brush. This will make the darkest shades appear as a wash of colour and is a great way to experiment with shades which you are not normally inspired to try.

POLISH WORK
To create new nail colour combinations you can try layering different polishes. Apply intense, deeper colours as the base coat and then add a sheer or iridescent top coat. Great colour ways are red with gold, purple with silver, and fuchsia with iridescent ivory. Alternatively, try adding different colours to half-used bottles of polish and shake well to mix.

FOUNDATION FIXES
As the seasons change, your foundation requirements are likely to differ. In summer, if your foundation is too thick, dilute with moisturizer. In winter, if your foundation does not offer sufficient coverage, mix with a small amount of super-fine powder to thicken it. Alternatively, mix concealer and foundation together, then smooth on.

GLISTENING SKIN
Add a small amount of silver powder (crush a pressed eyeshadow, using the flat side of a ruler) to loose face powder. Blend together and dust on to shoulders or parts of the body that may be revealed when you are wearing cut-away clothing to give the skin luminosity. Alternatively, mix foundation containing light-reflecting particles with body moisturizer.

BEAUTY INTELLIGENCE

If your eyes need brightening, it is a good idea to use sheer, enlivening shades of creamy beige, iridescent pearl, soft lilac or see-through wine eye colour.

If you don't have your concealer to hand, you can always use a brush dipped in foundation in order to cover any unsightly blemishes or under-eye circles.

You should always avoid using concealers that have either pink or orange undertones as they will only highlight rather than hide any imperfections or discolorations.

If you want your blusher to look really natural once you have applied it, you need to choose a shade that mimics your skin colour when you blush naturally.

If you want to look well groomed but not heavily made-up, ensure that you have no harsh make-up lines round the eyes. The secret as always is to blend thoroughly.

For blondes and those with fair hair, brown mascara is a more natural-looking option than black and if more definition is required a brown/black variety is suitable.

If you don't want to wear any make-up, try sweeping a large brush loaded with bronzing powder over your skin to create a healthy-looking golden finish.

You will get more mileage from your lipstick if you apply it with a lip brush. It is estimated that this way there are some twenty or so more applications to be had.

If you want to wear a really pale shade of eyeshadow, try adding definition to the eyes with a pencil and mascara to avoid the chance of looking washed out.

The tone of your skin will change with the seasons, so adapt the colour of your foundation to suit by adding light or dark powder to subtly warm it or cool it down.

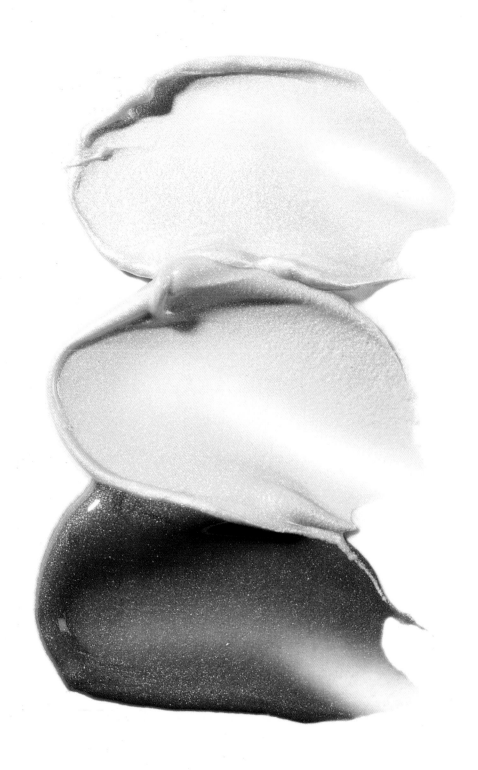

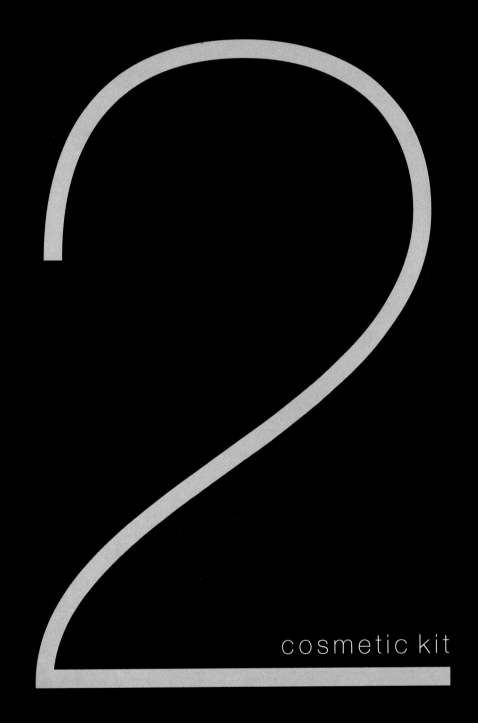

2 cosmetic kit

Choosing the right cosmetic implements will make all the difference between looking unkempt and looking well groomed. To achieve and then maintain your optimum appearance, you don't need to be a beauty professional. It is quite simply a case of finding the tools of the trade that are most suited to your own particular beauty needs.

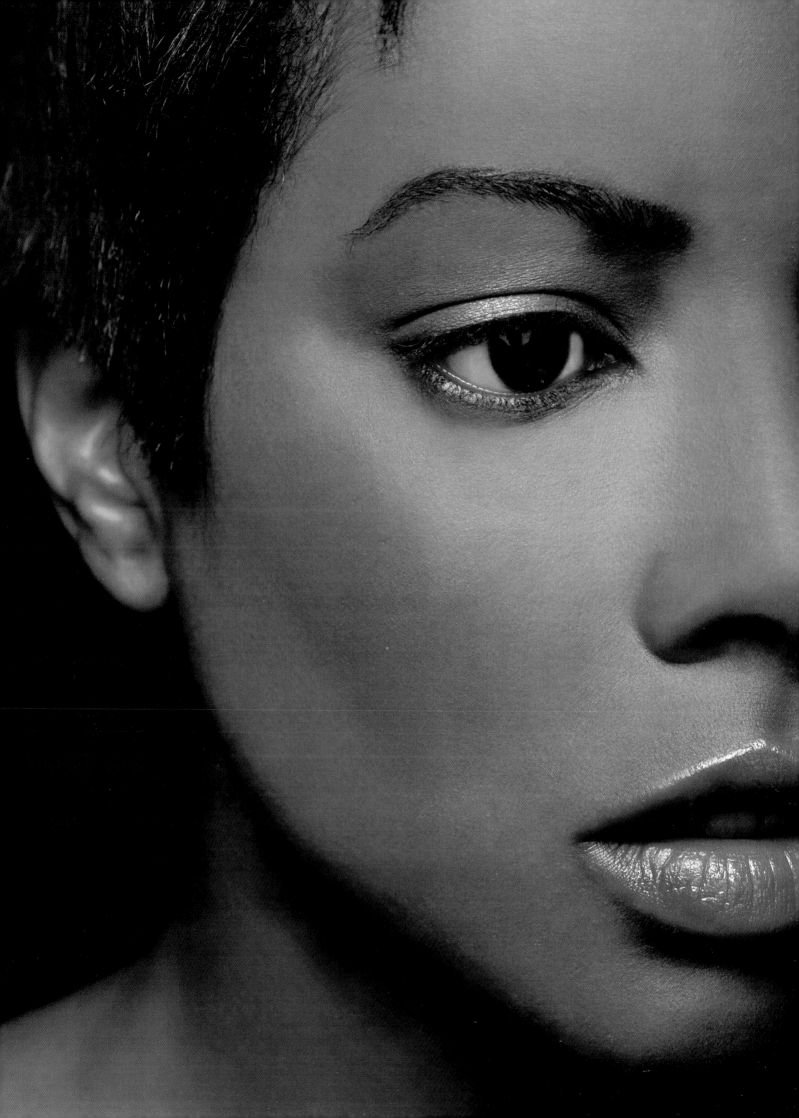

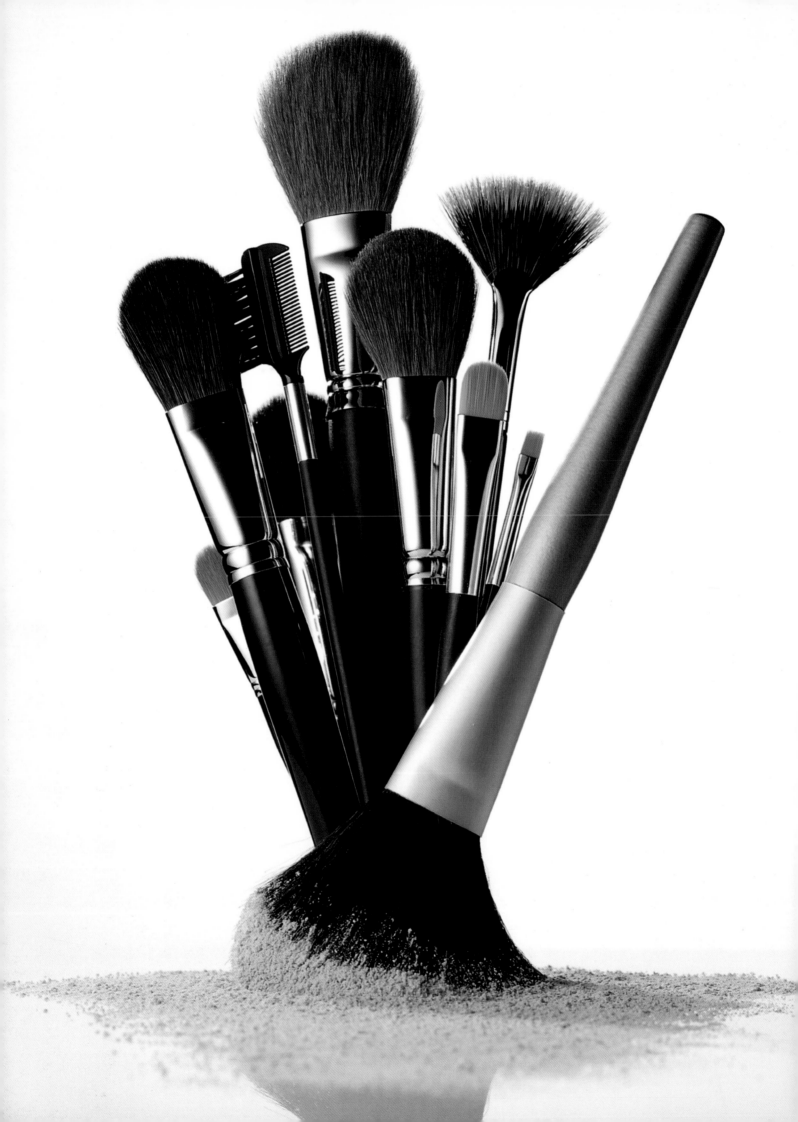

BRUSH WORKS

CHOOSING BRUSHES You don't need to arm yourself with every conceivable brush to perfect make-up application. In fact, you may prefer to apply some cosmetics with your fingertips or with the applicators provided. However, if you have trouble applying make-up, the right brushes can make all the difference. Knowing which ones to select and how to judge their quality can be daunting tasks. Make-up artists always advise investing in a set of good-quality brushes. Price usually gives some indication of quality, but when you're buying a brush you should also take into account how the bristles feel: too soft and they will not pick up and deposit colour correctly; too prickly and they will irritate and possibly pierce the skin.

QUALITY CONTROL You can test the quality of a brush by running it over the back of your hand. If the bristles all move in the same direction, this is a good sign. However, if they splay on the skin, this indicates that the brush will offer little control, resulting in haphazard application. Also look at how the bristles shed. It is quite normal for new brushes to lose a few bristles, but if the loss is excessive this can indicate poor quality. Try gently pulling at the bristles: if a mound comes away in your hand, do not buy the brush. Make sure the handle of the brush feels comfortable to the touch and fits well in your hand. And think about the look you are hoping to achieve: brushes which are soft and do not have a lot of control are ideal for quick, easy application, while those which are compact and have much tighter bristles are ideal for precision application.

NATURAL VS SYNTHETIC There has been much debate over the years on the relative merits of using synthetic and real hair (the animals aren't made to suffer in any way in the process) for bristles in make-up brushes. The best-quality bristles come from goats, sables and blue squirrels, but synthetic bristles are much cheaper and can offer good results.

WHAT TO LOOK FOR To disguise pimples and imperfections with concealer, opt for a synthetic-bristled brush which is narrow and has a flat, square tip. To apply powder, look for a soft-bristled, large brush which can be swept over the face in a couple of strokes. This can also be used to apply bronzing powder. To dust on powder blusher, use brushes which are tapered at the sides and have a rounded tip; they have been designed specifically to contour and sculpt the cheekbones without leaving streaks of colour. For filling sparse brows or shading and shaping the brows, look for a coarse-bristled brush that has a square or slant-edged tip. For applying eyeshadow, although sponge-tipped applicators are easy to control and make shading the eyelids a simple task, ensuring that colour is quite intense, you could equally well use a soft-bristled brush with tapered sides and a rounded tip. This will help you create a more natural-looking, sheer finish than is possible with a sponge-tipped applicator. For painting on eyeliner, choose a small, fine-tipped brush which is tapered to a point for precision lining. To shade and define the lips, look for a brush similar in shape to a concealer brush. When choosing a lip brush, go for one with firm bristles which is tapered to a flat, square tip. This will be ideal for outlining and shading the lips.

EXPERT ADVICE Customize your make-up brushes to suit your needs. You can use a pair of scissors and taper the ends of brushes so they mould to your features. For example, you can give an eyeshadow brush a slant-edged finish so it makes defining the socket line of the eyes an easier task; cut a coarse-bristled brush to a blunt finish and use as a brow shader; and transform a lip liner into a fine-tipped eyeliner brush.

GROOMING IMPLEMENTS

TWEEZERS are an essential implement for keeping your brows in trim. For plucking, choose a pair of long-handled, easy-to-hold ones with a slant edge to grip hairs effectively. For easing out ingrown hairs or splinters, go for tweezers with a fine point, but use them carefully as the sharp point can be lethal.

SCISSORS should be a staple of any cosmetic kit for cutting nails and trimming unruly brows. Scissors with curved ends are suitable for shaping fingernails, while scissors with straight edges are good for cutting toenails and creating a square finish. To prolong their life, make sure you dry scissors thoroughly if they get wet and store them in a protective case.

PENCIL SHARPENERS don't have to be a costly investment. Art supply shops have inexpensive ones which are suitable for most cosmetic pencils. Apart from keeping the points of liners and definers in shape, regular sharpening will help to ensure that they are clean and so prevent the spread of germs and bacteria.

COTTON BUDS are a must in your make-up kit in order to rectify any number of problems that might arise, such as flaking mascara, smudged eyeliner or feathered lipstick. For reasons of hygiene, you should buy them individually wrapped.

MAKE-UP SPONGES are not strictly necessary for applying foundation – you may prefer to smooth it on with your fingertips – but if you want to use a sponge, you should look for a triangular latex wedge. These are available from professional make-up shops and are perfectly shaped to work around the nose or sweep under the eyes.

EYELASH CURLERS should have a place in any cosmetic kit as they will keep the lashes in good shape. When you curl your lashes, it will instantly make you appear more awake and strengthen the eyes. Make-up artists recommend that you gently heat the ends of metal lash curlers with a hairdryer before using them, to literally set the lashes in place. Just be careful not to burn the tender skin around the eyes.

POWDER PUFFS might not be vital but they do make applying powder something of a treat. Goose-down powder puffs feel great on the skin but they can overload the complexion with powder. For a more natural finish, make-up artists recommend using velour powder puffs to press powder into the skin, especially around the nose, on the chin and on the forehead – all areas that are prone to excessive shine.

BROW BRUSH & LASH COMB is a dual-purpose product which is handy for achieving a well-groomed finish even if you're not wearing make-up. A lash comb will help if your mascara clogs during application. Always plant the comb near the roots and gently push upwards as you drag it through the lashes to help define the natural curl. You can dip the edge of the brow brush in hair gel or moisturizer before running it through the brows to help keep them in place.

MAGNIFYING MIRRORS are helpful when plucking the eyebrows and checking that eyeliner is straight, imperfections are concealed and make-up is blended. Don't use while applying make-up, as they can distort your features.

TISSUES are always useful to have with you. Among their many roles, they can be called upon to blot lipstick, to deal with overloaded mascara wands or, when pressed into the skin after the application of foundation, to absorb any excess oil from the product which otherwise might go on to interfere with the staying power of your make-up base.

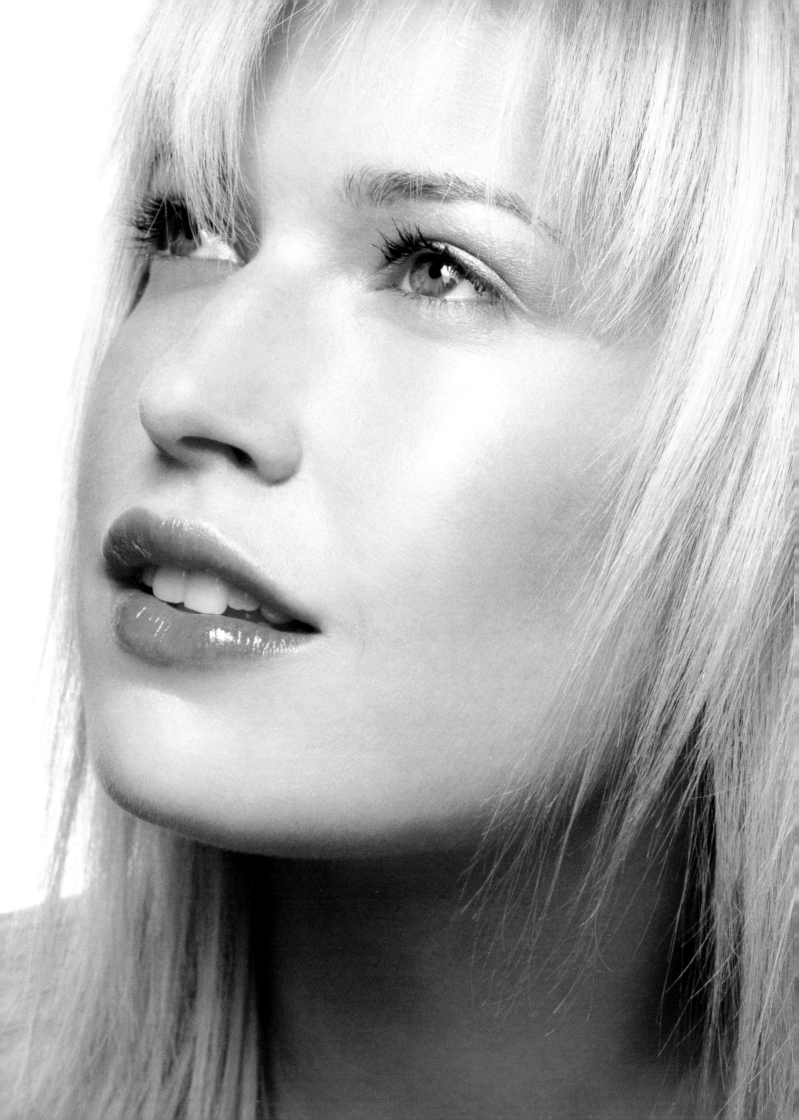

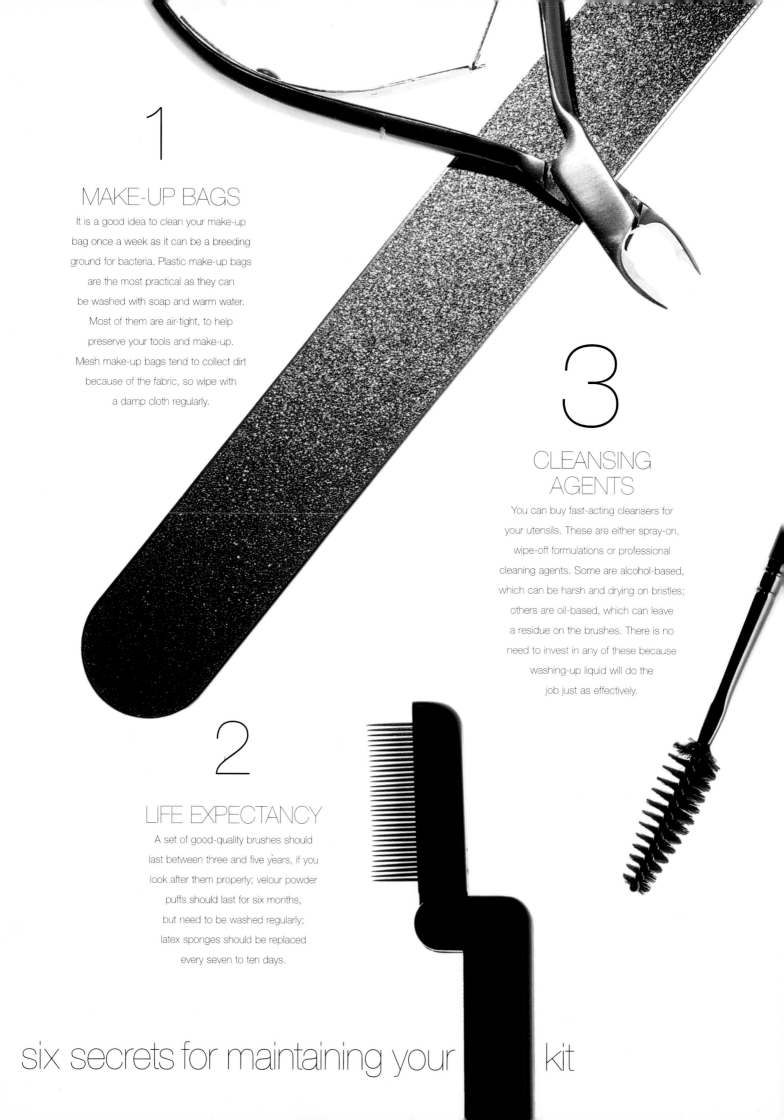

1

MAKE-UP BAGS

It is a good idea to clean your make-up
bag once a week as it can be a breeding
ground for bacteria. Plastic make-up bags
are the most practical as they can
be washed with soap and warm water.
Most of them are air-tight, to help
preserve your tools and make-up.
Mesh make-up bags tend to collect dirt
because of the fabric, so wipe with
a damp cloth regularly.

3

CLEANSING AGENTS

You can buy fast-acting cleansers for
your utensils. These are either spray-on,
wipe-off formulations or professional
cleaning agents. Some are alcohol-based,
which can be harsh and drying on bristles;
others are oil-based, which can leave
a residue on the brushes. There is no
need to invest in any of these because
washing-up liquid will do the
job just as effectively.

2

LIFE EXPECTANCY

A set of good-quality brushes should
last between three and five years, if you
look after them properly; velour powder
puffs should last for six months,
but need to be washed regularly;
latex sponges should be replaced
every seven to ten days.

six secrets for maintaining your kit

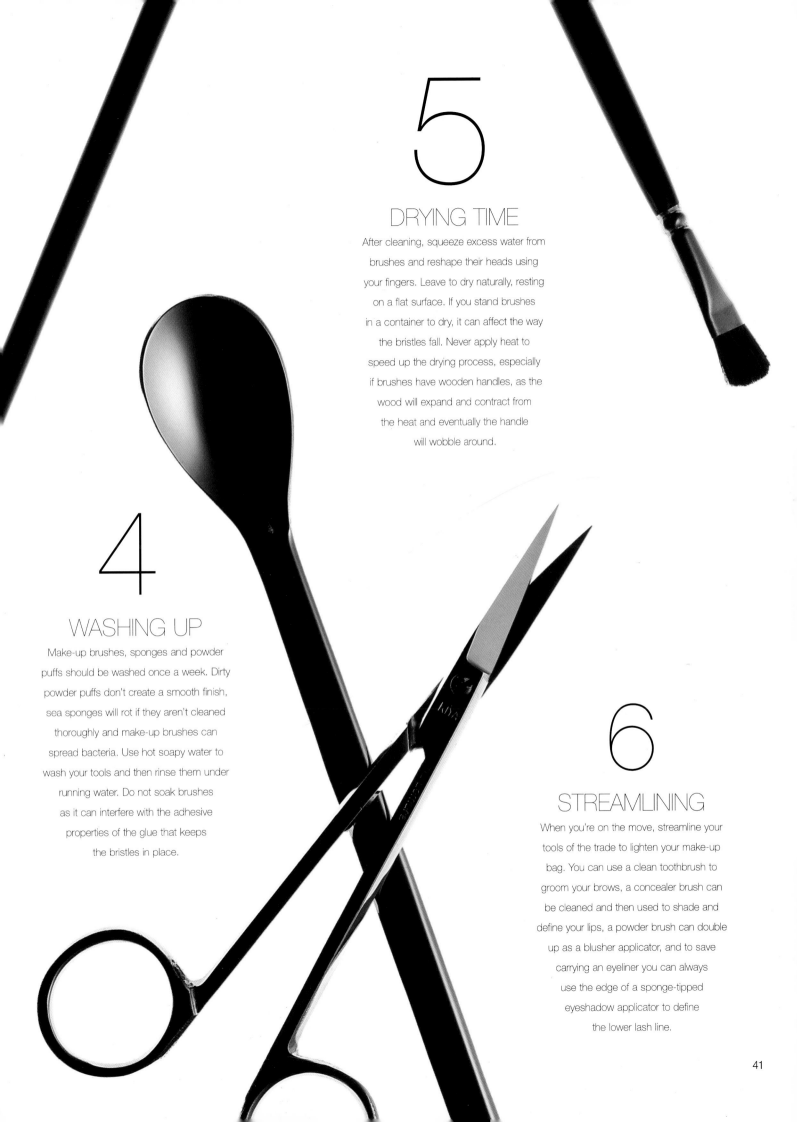

5

DRYING TIME

After cleaning, squeeze excess water from brushes and reshape their heads using your fingers. Leave to dry naturally, resting on a flat surface. If you stand brushes in a container to dry, it can affect the way the bristles fall. Never apply heat to speed up the drying process, especially if brushes have wooden handles, as the wood will expand and contract from the heat and eventually the handle will wobble around.

4

WASHING UP

Make-up brushes, sponges and powder puffs should be washed once a week. Dirty powder puffs don't create a smooth finish, sea sponges will rot if they aren't cleaned thoroughly and make-up brushes can spread bacteria. Use hot soapy water to wash your tools and then rinse them under running water. Do not soak brushes as it can interfere with the adhesive properties of the glue that keeps the bristles in place.

6

STREAMLINING

When you're on the move, streamline your tools of the trade to lighten your make-up bag. You can use a clean toothbrush to groom your brows, a concealer brush can be cleaned and then used to shade and define your lips, a powder brush can double up as a blusher applicator, and to save carrying an eyeliner you can always use the edge of a sponge-tipped eyeshadow applicator to define the lower lash line.

41

SHELF
LIFE

CONCEALER
will last for up to twelve months.

FACE POWDER
will last for up to two years.

FOUNDATION
water-based foundation will last for up to
twelve months, oil-based foundation will
last for up to about eighteen months.

EYE LINER
should be sharpened regularly and will
last for up to two years.

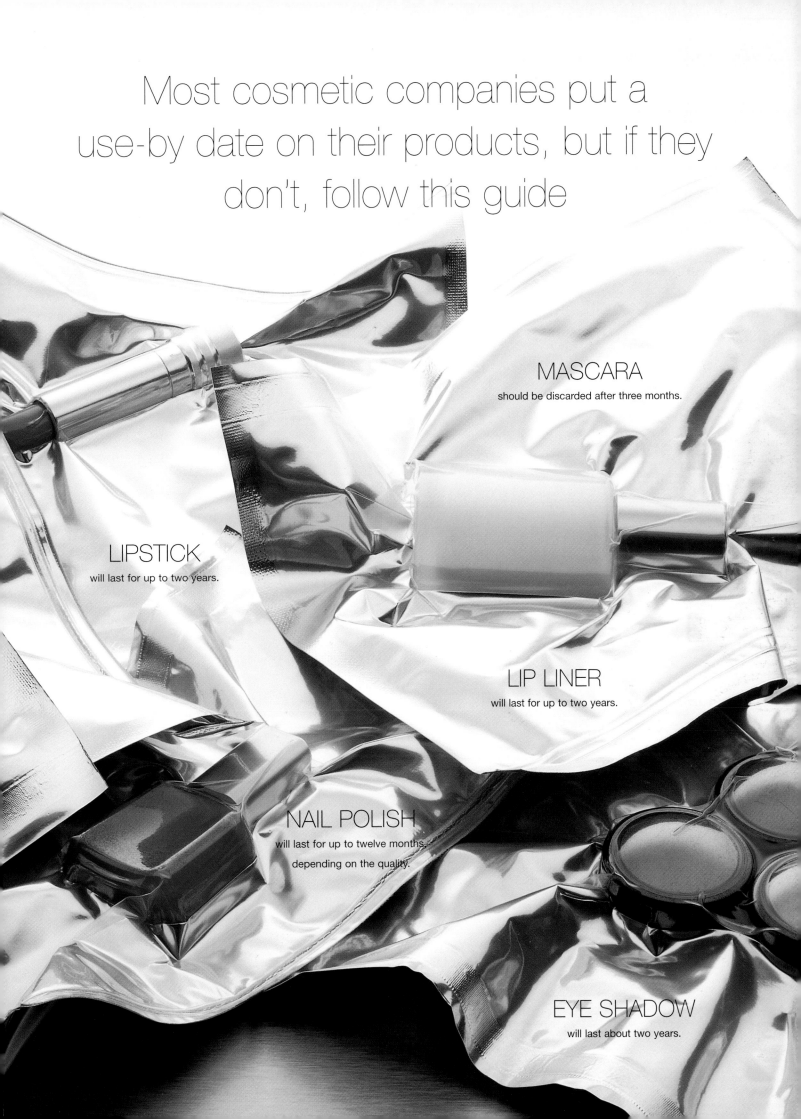

Most cosmetic companies put a use-by date on their products, but if they don't, follow this guide

MASCARA
should be discarded after three months.

LIPSTICK
will last for up to two years.

LIP LINER
will last for up to two years.

NAIL POLISH
will last for up to twelve months, depending on the quality.

EYE SHADOW
will last about two years.

SEASONALCHANGES

FOUNDATION

During the winter months opt for a creamy foundation which helps prevent skin from dehydrating, and when the heat is on during the summer months switch to an oil-free formulation. The skin produces more oil during the hot weather and so these formulations will work with the skin's natural balance. Lightweight, tinted moisturizers are also a good option.

POWDER

Any pressed or loose powder can be used all year round, but an oil-free powder is a better choice during the summer months as it will help keep unsightly oil secretions at bay. If you want a healthy glow, switch face powder with bronzing powder during the summer. Look for a bronzer which is laced with subtle shimmer to make your skin look luminous as well as healthy.

BLUSHER

Creamy formulations will melt into the skin and won't have a drying effect on the skin, making them ideal for winter wear; powder blusher can be a good option for the summer as it helps absorb surface oils. Try wearing lavender pink shades to brighten the pallor of winter complexions and in the summer choose soft peaches and burnished browns to warm the skin.

BASE

If you smooth on foundation only to find it looks slightly too dark for your skin tone, instead of removing and starting again, simply press translucent face powder into the skin to tone down the colour. Afterwards, if your skin looks too powdery, spray with a fine mist of water. If your foundation looks too pale after applying, warm it up by dusting the face with bronzing powder.

adapt your make-up bag to suit the season

COLOUR
Although there are no strict rules as to what you can and cannot wear, adapt your colour palette to suit the season. During the winter, if you look pale and washed out, warm the skin with soft corals and peaches or incorporate brighter shades into your make-up look. During the summer, coppers, burnished browns and golds will give the skin a flattering finish.

FORMULATIONS
During the summer, it is best to steer clear of make-up products which are creamy and prone to melt. When the heat is on, cheeks will be naturally rosy so there is no need to wear blusher. If your mascara has a tendency to flake and smudge under the eyes when it is hot, do not wear it – instead have your eyelashes tinted. Look for cosmetics with UV filters.

MASCARA
Mascara is a trans-seasonal item, so the only change you may wish to make is substituting your existing mascara with a waterproof formula during the summer months or when you go on holiday. Waterproof formulations can be drying on the lashes so coat them with a thin film of Vaseline as a conditioning treat at night, once a fortnight or when your lashes feel brittle.

LIPSTICK
For winter wear, look for a moisture-rich lipstick that will help protect the lips from chapping and dryness. Avoid wearing lipsticks which dry to a matt finish as they can have a dehydrating effect. During the summer, look for a lipstick with an in-built sunscreen to help protect against the sun's harmful UV rays. Sheer tints and lip glosses are ideal for summer wear.

BEAUTY INTELLIGENCE

1

Before tweezing the brows, cleanse the skin. If you cannot stand the pain of plucking, numb the area first with babies' teething gel or with an ice cube.

2

If your nail scissors are blunt or the edges of your tweezers have lost their grip, you can run sandpaper gently over the inner blunt edges to sharpen them.

3

Don't try to salvage nail polish that has dried out and gone hard by diluting it with nail polish remover. It will not solve the problem, so just throw it away.

4

Try not to lend make-up brushes to other people as this can spread infections. If you have no choice, always wash brushes thoroughly before reusing them.

5

When you're looking for make-up brushes, go first to art supply stores. You can pick up great brushes for half the price of those found in cosmetic shops.

When the bristles of your brushes start to become untidy and begin to fray, revamp them by using a pair of nail scissors to trim stray hairs back into shape.

6

7

You should never buff the nails after taking a bath or shower, because the cuticles will be too soft then and so damage might occur to the surrounding skin.

9

After plucking your eyebrows, do not apply any make-up for at least an hour. Tweezing before bed gives any irritation time to calm down while you're asleep.

After applying your moisturizer, you should always allow the skin to absorb it and settle for at least ten minutes before smoothing on any make-up preparations.

8

If you want to apply eyeshadow with a sponge-tipped applicator, don't try using those provided in the palettes as their size can make them hard to manoeuvre.

10

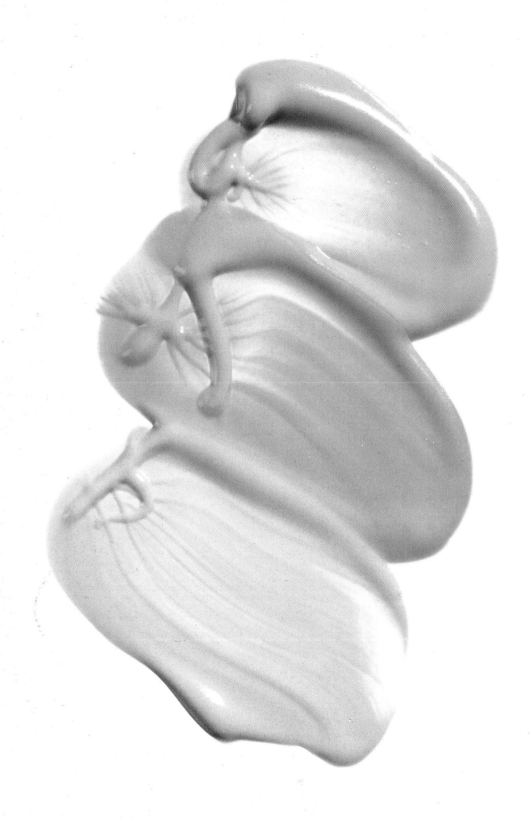

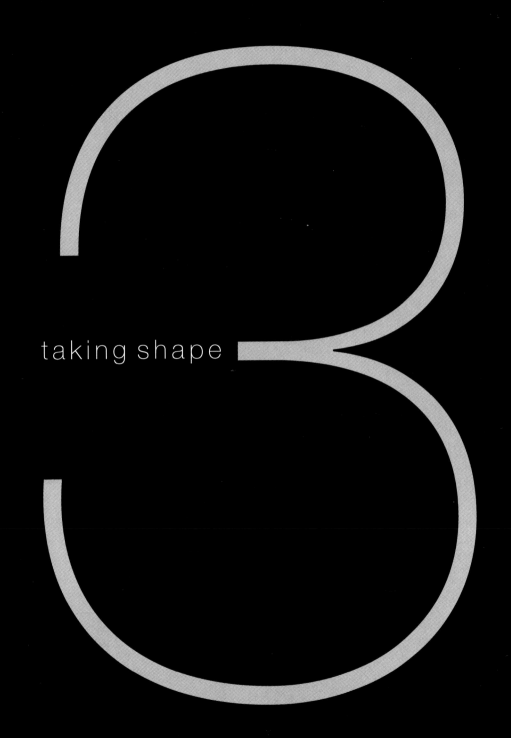

taking shape

In your ideal world maybe you imagine yourself genetically blessed with model-like looks, but the reality is that most of us have features which are not perfect. You may worry about having a prominent nose, small, deep-set eyes or uneven lips, but these are actually what gives your face its individuality, so try treating them as marks of beauty.

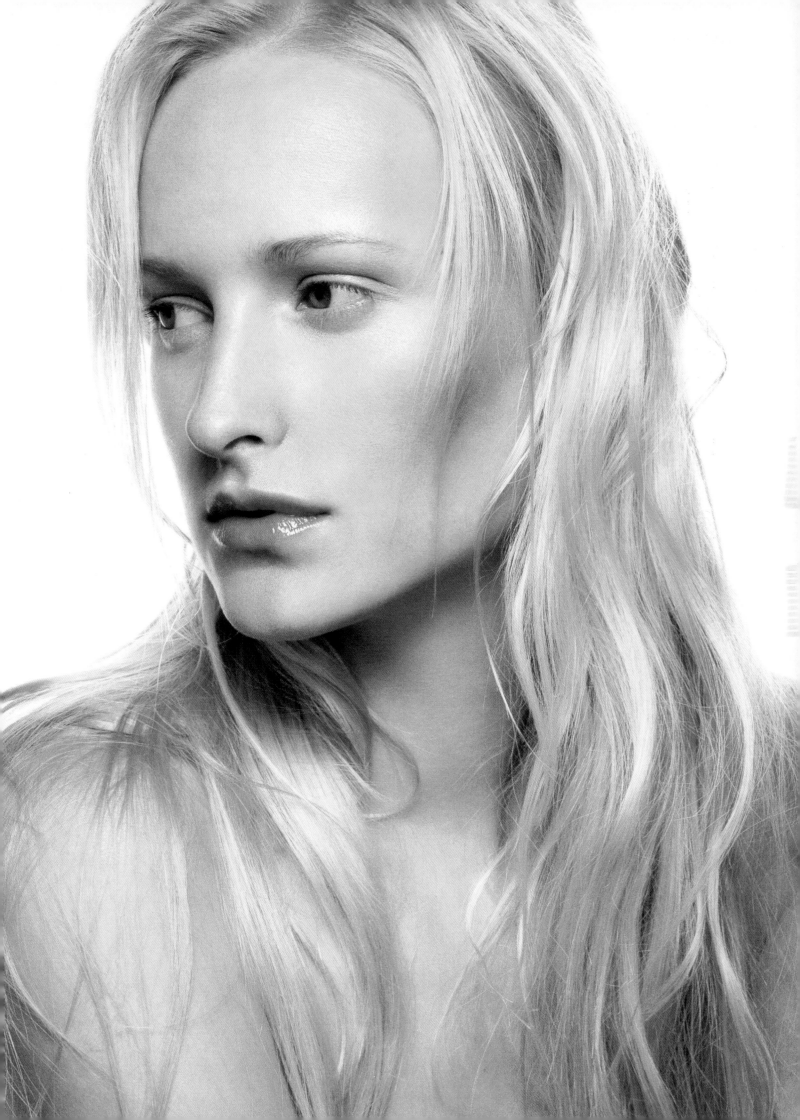

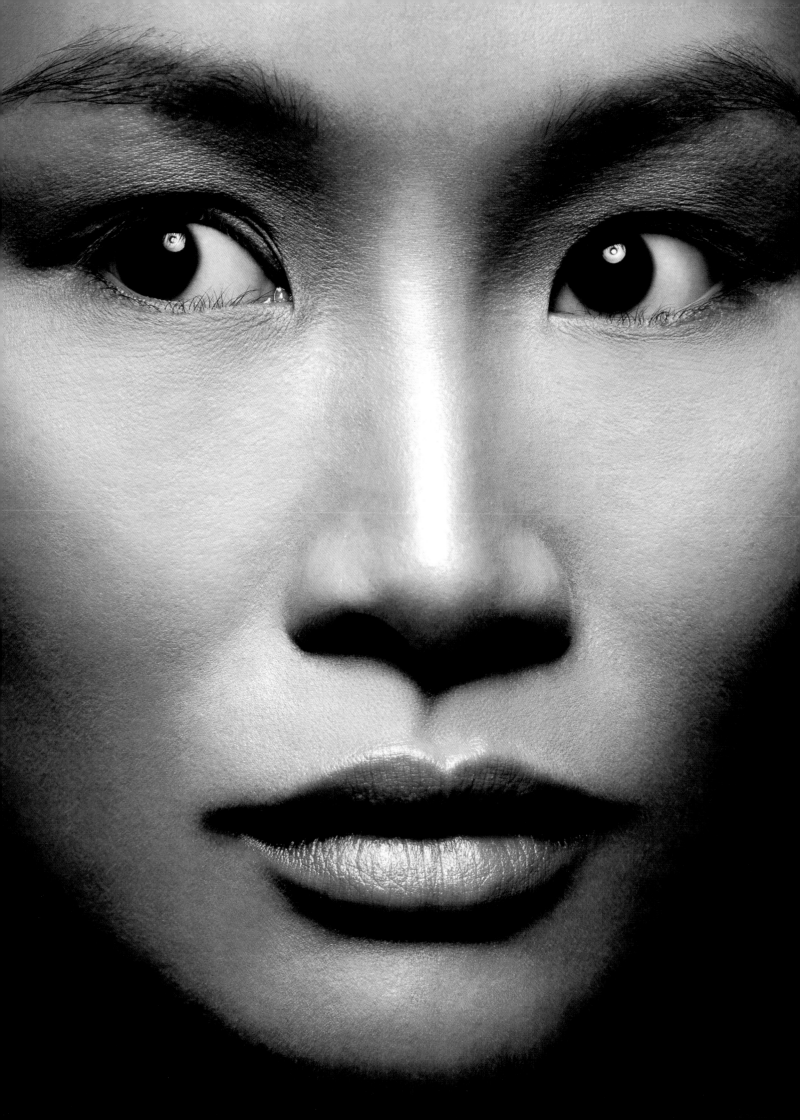

CHEEKBONES

If you don't have razor-sharp cheekbones, get to work contouring the face to create the illusion of a perfect shape and perfectly formed features that will bring out the structure of the face. Look for a face powder or blusher that echoes the natural shadows created under prominent bones, choosing a shade slightly darker than your foundation, such as a beige blusher. To get the contour in the correct place, gently suck in the cheeks and then apply right beneath the cheekbone. Blusher can also be added a little further up, actually on top of the cheekbone itself, if this is what you want.

ROUND FACE

Round faces, which are usually short and fairly wide with full cheeks and a rounded chin, have the advantage of always looking youthful. To make the most of your face, avoid accentuating the shape. Do not wear blusher on the cheek apples, but instead softly sculpt the cheekbones. Don't overdo it, or the results will look false and draw attention to your face. Avoid the kohl-rimmed look, apply eye colours to elongate the eyes and so balance the face. Your brow should be tapered towards the tip of the ear. If you wear glasses, slim down your face with square, rectangular or cat's-eye frames.

LONG FACE

Long faces usually have high cheekbones, a deep forehead and a strong, sharp or chiselled jawline. To balance a long face, do not make the arch of the eyebrow too extreme; rather, soften your features and keep your brow shape in a straight line which tapers towards the tip of the ear. Apply blusher to the cheek apples in small circular motions to create a rosy-cheeked effect and avoid softly sculpting the cheeks since this will only elongate the face. If you wear glasses, you should look for frames that are round or curved, because these will help to break up the narrow shape of the face.

HEART-SHAPED FACE

Wider around the forehead and curving down to a point, this kind of face can look very dainty and pretty. To enhance the overall shape, you should highlight the tip of the chin, using a pale shade of face powder or a subtle ivory highlighter. Work on the temples next, blending the colour into the hairline (you will need to be careful if you have blonde hair because the colour will show). Add blusher to the cheek hollows (the areas just below the cheekbone). If you have small features, you should strengthen the appearance of either the lips or the eyes with make-up to give the face increased definition.

SQUARE FACE

In order to take the edge off a square face, highlight the central strip of the face by dusting on an ivory-coloured eyeshadow or face powder, going down the forehead and nose to the tip of the chin. Using a face powder one shade darker than your existing colour, shade around the hairline, where visible, and then softly shade the extremities of your jawline. Apply blusher to the cheek apples in small circular motions. When grooming the brows, ensure that their ends curve towards the middle of the ear. If you wear glasses, look for thin frames in oval or round shapes as they will balance the face.

MOLES & FRECKLES

If you have a mole on your face, treat it as a striking feature. Make-up artists transform moles (or larger-than-life freckles) into beauty spots with waterproof definers. Simply shade the area with a black pencil. Examine any moles regularly. If you notice changes in colour, appearance or texture, seek expert advice. Do not pluck hairs from moles, but simply trim with nail scissors. If you try to cover freckles with foundation, they can look chalky, so instead show them off as part of a freshed-faced beauty look. Freckles and brown liver spots can be treated with a fade-out cream that contains hydroquinone.

DOUBLE CHIN

To make a double chin less obvious, use face powder one shade darker than normal to softly shade the chin area. This will create the illusion that it's receding, making it less obvious. Dab highlighter on the tip of the chin to brighten it. Make sure you blend thoroughly for a natural-looking finish. Give your neck and chin an invigorating massage every night while you are applying moisturizer. Placing your fingertips on one side of the throat and your thumb on the other side, gently rotate in small circular motions up and down the throat. Then, using the upper side of the hand, slap lightly under the chin area.

NOSE JOB

If you have a big nose and are self-conscious about the fact, wear a strong lip colour or make your eyes the focal point of your face with make-up, thus drawing attention away from the nose. To soften and streamline the bridge of the nose, dust on a light taupe shade of matt eyeshadow, working down either side of the bridge of your nose and then up towards the eyebrows. To take any hard edge off the nose, shade the tip before applying a rosy beige cheek or eye colour on the underside and between the nostrils. You'll find that this will also help if you want to make a long nose appear slightly shorter.

TOOTH TACTICS

If you are conscious that you do not have perfect teeth, wearing brightly coloured or strong shades of lipstick can draw attention to the mouth. If tooth enamel is stained, which can occur from the tannin in tea, the caffeine in drinks, eating certain foods and smoking, have your teeth professionally cleaned and polished by a dental hygienist at least twice a year. For at-home stain relief, rub the peel from a lemon over the teeth and then rinse with water. Avoid frosted peach and creamy beige tones of lipstick, as these have a tendency to make your teeth appear an unsightly shade of yellow.

FACIAL HAIR

Excessive facial hair can either be a hereditary condition or the result of a hormone imbalance. If the condition is severe, contact your GP and have a blood test to detect imbalances and receive treatment. There are three main methods to deal with the problem: waxing, which removes hairs for up to six weeks; electrolysis, which uses a needle to target each hair individually, zapping it at the roots (the drawback is that a course of treatments is required to permanently remove them all); and laser treatment, which targets hair at the roots with immediate results, although maintenance sessions are required.

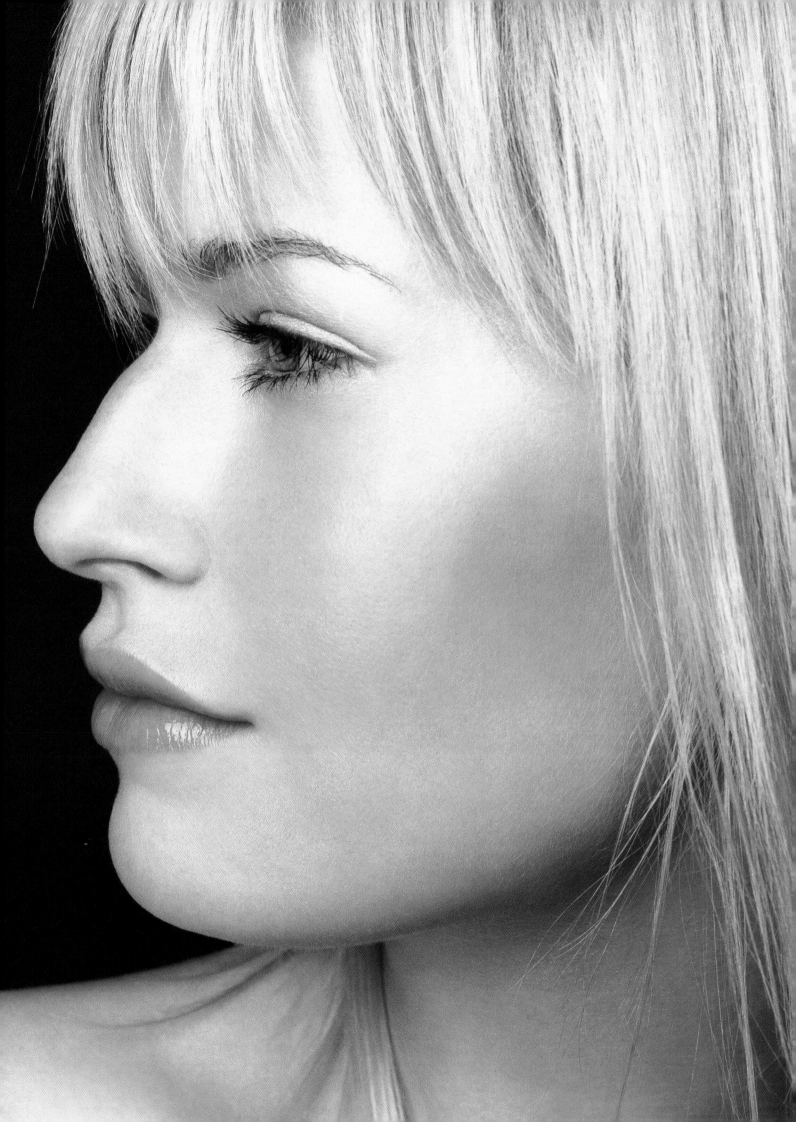

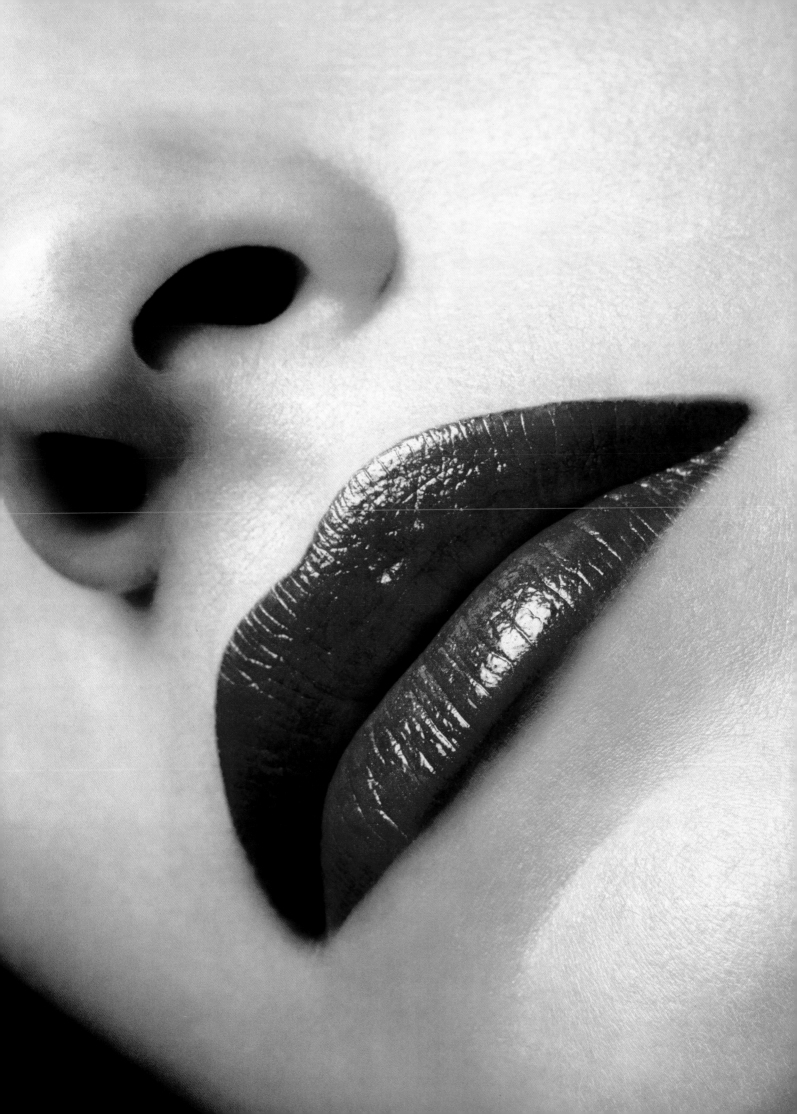

LIP SHAPES

THIN LIPS There is no point trying to draw a line outside your natural lip line in an attempt to make your lips appear bigger. It will just look a mess and unnatural. Instead, use lip liner to add extra curve to thin lips and to accentuate the natural lip line. To create the illusion of fullness, wear light- to medium-toned lipsticks and experiment with lip gloss to make the lips appear larger than they really are. Make-up artists recommend that, after applying lip colour, you dab lip gloss on to the centre of the lower lip, then purse the lips together. This will create the illusion of all-over gloss while ensuring the colour stays in place longer. Always avoid wearing bright reds or very dark lip colours because they can give thin lips a sultry, mean appearance.

FULL LIPS If you have full, luscious lips, make the most of them and paint on a bold shade of lipstick – remember, many women pay good money to have their lips plumped up with implants. However, for those who want to play down fullness, skip lip liner and wear paler shades of lipstick. Avoid gloss, as it only accentuates fullness; matt is a better option. To draw attention away from the lips, wear a hint of colour and then use make-up to ensure your eyes are the focal point of your face.

UNEVEN LIPS It is very common to have thinner top lips and fuller bottom lips – this is true for over 90 per cent of women. To achieve better balance, outline the outside edge of the top lip and then keep the line within the natural shape of the lower lip. Use a lighter shade of lipstick on the upper lip and then a slightly darker shade of the same colour on the fuller lip. Purse the lips together after application. This should create a very subtle difference in colour and will help address the problem. If in your case it is the bottom lip that's thinner than the top one, reverse the tonal colour combination just described.

WIDE LIPS To draw attention away from the width of the lips, concentrate the intensity of the colour on the central part, gradually fading outwards. Do not use liner to accentuate the overall shape of the lips but instead use it to emphasize your Cupid's bow, thus adding extra height to the lips. After applying colour, dab on silver gloss to the centre of the lower lip, over the lipstick. Apart from creating an interesting finish, this will make more of your pout, in the process directing attention to the centre of your mouth and away from the edges of your lips.

SMALL LIPS Medium-toned lipsticks will look very attractive on small lips, whereas dark, strong shades are not suitable. Experiment with a range of different textures to make the most of small lips, looking especially for shimmery, glossy or sheer tints in brighter colours. To accentuate lips, after applying your lipstick get to work with a lip pencil on the outer corners of the mouth. Use a colour that is slightly darker than your lipstick and shade the outer sections of the upper and lower lips. Blend in with your lipstick, using your fingertip or a make-up brush. This will give your lips improved definition, which in turn will create the illusion that they are bigger than they in reality are.

DOWN-TURNED LIPS You can lift a down-turned mouth by applying concealer around the outer edges of the lips, since this is where a natural shadow may be cast. This will instantly highlight the area and so lift the mouth. Do not apply dark colours, especially around the outer corners of the lips, and do not use lip liner to trace the natural contour of the lips, both of which will only accentuate the lips' natural droop. Opt instead for paler shades on the outer corners of the lips, focusing the intensity of the colour on the central zone. You should always go for sheer textures to get the very best results.

EYE SHAPES

SMALL EYES This shape is characterized by a short distance between the upper and lower lashes. To open the eyes up, experiment with light shades of eyeshadow. Avoid dark colours as they will make the eyes appear even smaller. Sweep a wash of colour in a light shade over the eyelid to enlarge and illuminate the eyes, then shade the outer corner of the lid and the socket line with a slightly darker shade. Define the outer corners of the upper and lower eye with a pencil, tapering the line outwards to elongate the eyes. Add a subtle highlight to the top of the brow bone and apply lots of mascara to open the eyes up. Keep the brows well groomed to ensure that there are no stray hairs on the brow area, as this can make the eye space appear even smaller.

WIDE-SET A sense of innocence always accompanies wide-set eyes, but if this is not the effect you want, to make them appear closer together focus colour and definer on the inner corners of the eyes. Start off by sweeping a light colour wash over the eye area, then dust on a medium colour on the inner half of the eyelid before blending outwards to create a natural finish. Next you need to contour the socket line, using a darker shade. Concentrate intensity on the inner half of the socket and softly fade outwards. Take eyeliner from the inner corner to the middle of the eye and then blend outwards. Make sure that the lashes on the inside of the eye are coated with sufficient mascara to create the illusion of decreased distance.

CLOSE-SET If your eyes are less than one eye-length apart, create the illusion of added width by keeping the inner corners of the eyes light and bright and then shading the outer corners. Sweep a light shade across the eyelid before dusting a medium shade on to the outer half of the eyelid. Add darker eyeshadow to the outer corner of the socket line. With an eyeliner, define from the middle of the top and bottom lash line, extending and tapering up and out, about 6mm past the outer corner of the eyes. Concentrate mascara on the outer lashes.

DEEP-SET If you have deep-set eyes, your brow bone will be more prominent than your eyelid, so you'll want to make the eyelid more pronounced and create a balance between the upper and lower lids. Use a light- to medium-toned shadow over the entire eyelid, then a slightly darker shade above the eye crease to play down the brow bone. Define the upper lash line with a pencil, keeping the line fine on the inner corner of the eyes and getting thicker as you reach the middle of the eyelid, tapering it out. Repeat on the lower lash line, smudging for a neutral effect. Highlight the brow bone and add several coats of mascara. For a more dramatic effect, choose intense shades of neutral colours rather than the darker shades of eyeshadow.

VANISHING LID The eyelids of oriental women are invisible when their eyes are open, so for definition sweep a medium-toned eyeshadow over the eyelid and brow area. Dust under the brow with pale highlighter to bring out the brow bone and add contrast to the eyes. Use a pencil eyeliner, with the line very fine and natural-looking. Work along upper and lower lash lines, keeping the bottom line soft. Alternatively, instead of eyeshadow, paint on a thick smoky line along the upper lash line and under the eye. Oriental eyelashes can be thin, so define with a lash-building mascara.

DROOPY EYES Down-turned eyes need to be lifted to avoid looking sad and tired. Keep the attention on the eyelids rather than the lash lines. Apply eyeshadow on the outer corner of the eyelid, extending the colour up and out in a feline shape. Add highlighter to the brow bone using a very light shade. Avoid using eyeliner as it will trace the droopy contour. Use mascara, concentrating on the lashes at the inner corner of the eyes – this will have a 'lifting' effect. Alternatively, try a smudge of silver on the inner corners of the eyes to brighten and again to lift.

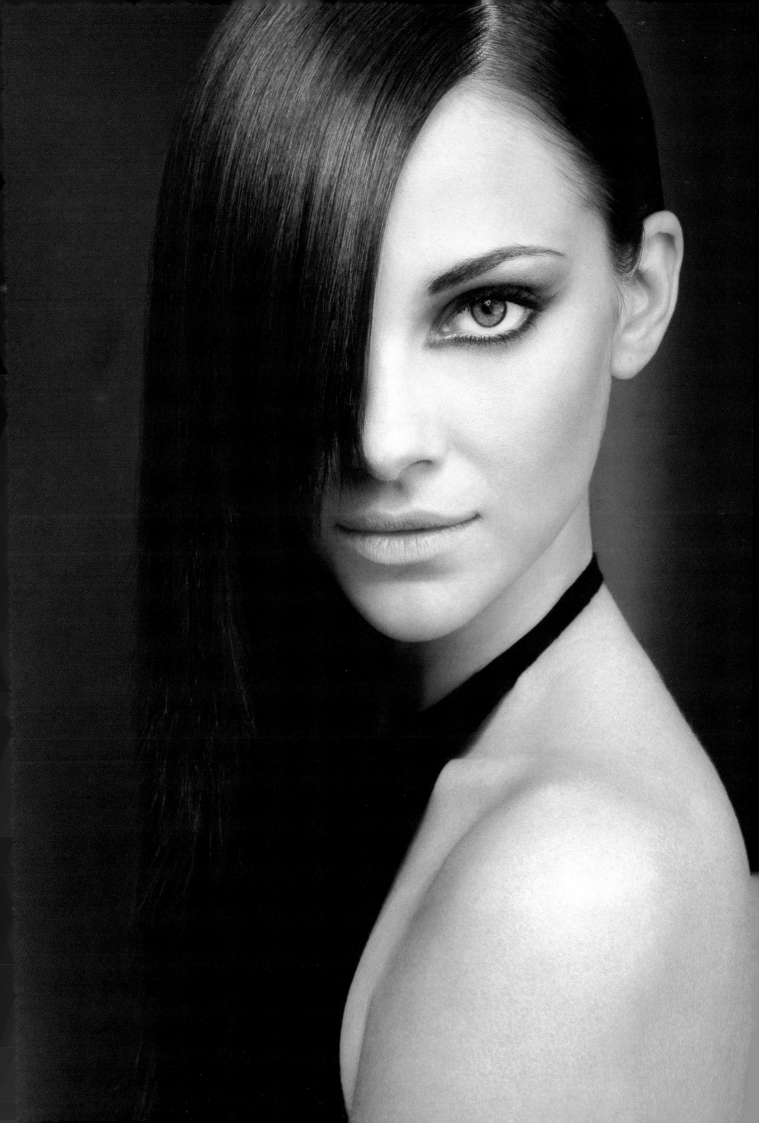

FOUNDATION

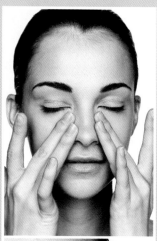

1. Apply compact foundation with a sponge; apply liquid formulas with your fingertips or a sponge. There is absolutely no need to whitewash the complexion with foundation. Instead you should simply dot it where it is really needed, such as areas of uneven skin tone, open pores and broken blood vessels.

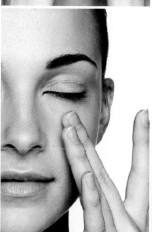

2. Ensure that coverage is even and blend foundation thoroughly. Work over the jawline and down the neck, so it is not possible to see where your foundation starts and finishes.

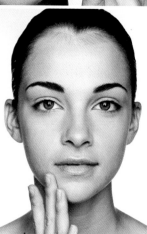

3. Using a brush or your fingertips, dab concealer under the eyes and then disguise any imperfections. To cover pimples, apply the concealer with a small brush, concentrating on the centre of the imperfection and then feathering slowly outwards.

4. After applying foundation, blot the complexion with a tissue to remove any excess oil in the product, which can interfere with the staying power of your base. To ensure you have no tell-tale application marks, examine your face with a magnifying mirror.

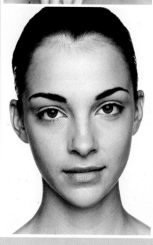

POWDER

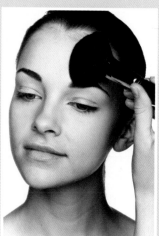

1. Use loose or pressed powder to set your make-up base. Always dust powder on to the skin in downward strokes as this prevents particles of powder getting trapped under superfluous facial hairs and creates an even finish.

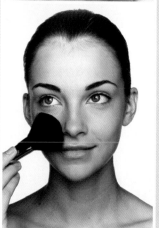

2. You do not need to apply powder all over the face. Concentrate on areas prone to shine, such as the nose, the chin and the forehead. Apply sparingly and aim to give your skin a seemingly unmade-up finish.

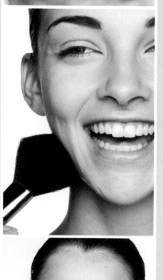

3. When retouching powder, blot the skin with a tissue and then dust the complexion with face powder. This will remove any build-up of product, which can combine with the skin's natural oils to give a clogged and unflattering finish.

4. Finally, when you have applied your powder, spray the face with a fine mist of water or toner. Gently press a tissue into the complexion using your fingertips and then smoothly lift it off. This will ensure you are left with a natural-looking finish which is not too powdery.

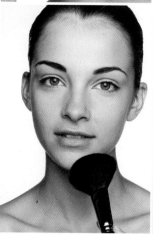

EYESHADOW

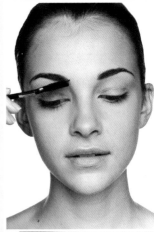

1. The simplest and most effective way to define the eyes is to use what is known as the three-step method of application. Select three eyeshadows in different shades from the same colour family: for example, a pale ivory, a medium terracotta and a good deep bronze.

2. Use the darkest shade to colour the eyelid. Work outwards from the inner corner of the lid. Do not take the colour right up into the socket line, but rather apply it in small sweeping strokes all over the eyelid.

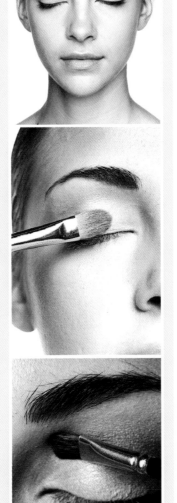

3. Next, using the medium-tone eyeshadow, shade the socket line, working out from the inner corner. Try raising your eyebrows to gently lift the eyes, as this should make it easier for you to define the line.

4. Finish off by using the palest shade to add a touch of colour to the brow bone. Use a magnifying mirror to check what you have done. If further blending is required, use your fingertips or work over the eye with a small, clean make-up brush to get the effect you want.

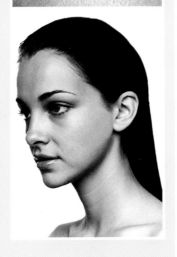

BROW DEFINERS

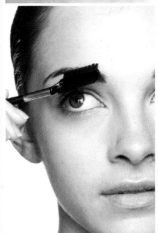

1. Defining the eyebrows helps to frame the face. Before defining, brush through with a brow comb to remove any stray hairs or particles of foundation and face powder. Initially brush through in the opposite direction to the natural hair-growth, and then rebrush into shape.

2. Use a brow definer in a shade that complements your brow colour. To define with a pencil, do not draw on one line over each eyebrow. Instead, create a natural-looking finish by applying in small feathered strokes (no longer than the average length of a brow hair). Start at the inner corner of the brow and gradually taper outwards.

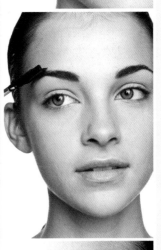

3. Then rub over the brows with a brush or your fingertip to ensure they don't look too heavily made up. If you've been heavy-handed, use a moist cotton bud and gently roll over the brow to lift off any excess.

4. To add the final touches, you can slick the brows down with a thin film of Vaseline. This will keep them in place and create a high-shine finish.

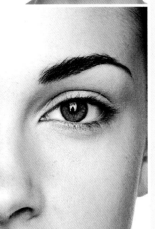

MASCARA

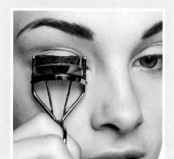

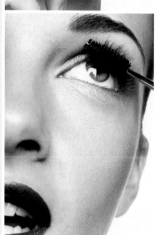

1. To give your lashes the best definition possible, you should use eyelash curlers before applying mascara. You might also want to wipe the mascara wand first with a tissue in order to remove any excess product if it is overloaded.

2. Then plant the wand into the eyelashes, close to the roots, and gradually pull through, while gently working the brush back and forth. As well as applying the mascara, this will also help reinforce the curl.

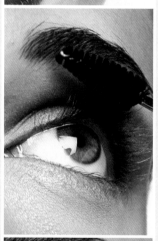

3. Work through the eyelashes with a lash comb to separate and define. Make sure that the fine wispy lashes on the outer corners of the eyes have picked up sufficient mascara. If they haven't, use the tip of the wand to define these stragglers.

4. Once the first coat of mascara is dry (this will normally take about sixty seconds), apply a top coat. Two fine coats will always look much more professional than one heavy-handed application. Finally, once both coats are dry, brush through again with a lash comb if required.

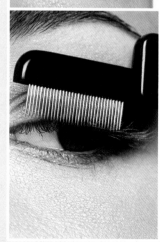

LIP DEFINERS

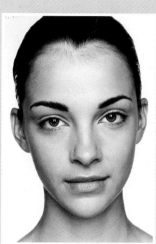

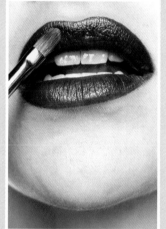

1. Before applying lip liner, you should always prime your lips with foundation in order to create a base for the lipstick. Look for an oil-free or a long-lasting foundation as this will improve the staying power of your lip colour. If your lips are prone to dryness, try coating them with a thin film of non-greasy lip balm before you smooth on your foundation.

2. Do not attempt to draw on one unbroken line round the lips. Unless you are a real professional, the chances are that your line will be uneven, and will also look dated and unnatural. Instead, for the best results, try applying the liner in small feathered strokes around the lips.

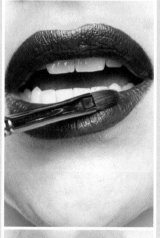

3. Then work over the entire lip area with lip liner, shading the lower and upper lips. Choose a shade similar to your natural lip colour or one to complement your choice of lipstick.

4. Finish by working over with a lip brush to blend thoroughly so as not to leave any harsh lines. If you don't want to wear lipstick as a top coat, you could slick on lip gloss instead.

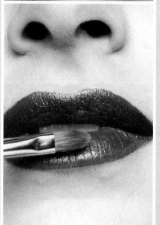

LIPSTICK

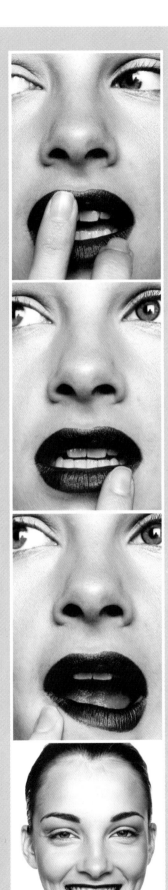

1. Ideally you should apply lipstick with a brush. Start at the outer corners of the lower lip and then fill in the central area. Once you are satisfied with the results, repeat this process on the upper lip. Finish by blotting your lips gently with a tissue to remove any excess product.

2. Reapply lipstick and then repeat the process of blotting with a tissue and coating with lipstick several times. If you want to be sure that your lipstick will really stay put, press a velour powder puff into your lips, then add one final coat of lipstick.

3. For a more dramatic look, dab a bright lip colour that corresponds to your base shade on to the centre of the upper and lower lips, then purse the lips together. You'll find this will create a wearable, 'bee-stung' look.

4. Add the finishing touches by dabbing lip gloss on to the centre of the lower lip. This will create the illusion of all-over gloss and also ensure that the gloss stays put and doesn't spoil the overall effect by bleeding into the surrounding skin.

BLUSHER

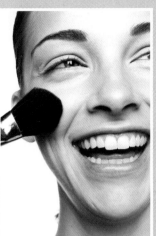

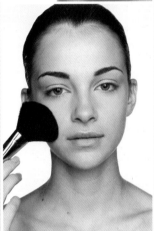

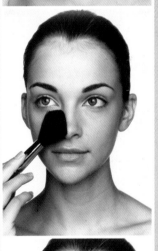

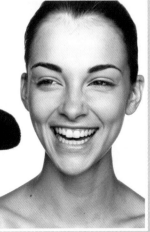

1. Before you apply your powder blusher, blow on a loaded blusher brush in order to remove any excess product. If you overdo things with the blusher, you can tone down the colour by dusting with translucent powder or blotting with a damp make-up sponge.

2. To softly sculpt the cheekbones, apply your blusher in small circular motions, working carefully down the cheekbone. This will ensure that you are left with a natural-looking finish instead of unsightly stripes of colour.

3. In order to define your cheek apples, locate the cheekbone and dab on colour. Literally massage it into the skin, again working in small circular motions, and this will give your skin a healthy flush of colour.

4. If you would like to add a flattering highlight to your cheeks, use your fingertips to dab shimmering ivory highlighter on to the top of the cheekbone. Working away from the eyes, blend downwards. You want to create a soft, subtle effect, so try to apply the highlighter sparingly.

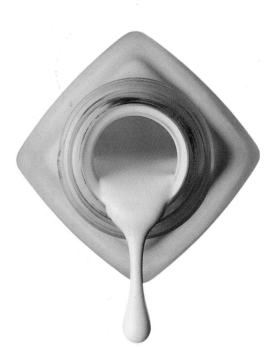

2

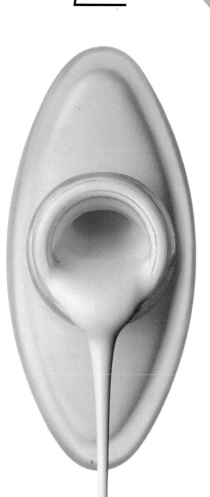

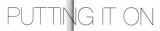

1

COLOUR CORRECTORS

Applied under foundation, colour-corrective creams or concealers mask imperfections that can't be disguised with standard concealer. Designed to even out skin tone, brighten lifeless-looking complexions, hide broken blood vessels and revive sallow skins, they work by counteracting the opposite hue on the colour wheel.

COLOUR CHOICE

Select a colour to tackle your problem: pale blue-green takes the redness out of flushed cheeks, sunburn or networks of thread veins; lilac revives tired, sallow skin and adds radiance in harsh lights; blue works wonders with dark patches on pale complexions and tones down mild redness around the base of the nose and on the cheeks; apricot is a general pick-me-up for dull skin; white gives luminosity and balances discoloured and mottled skin.

PUTTING IT ON

Apply these colour-corrective primers on top of moisturizer and under foundation. Keep coverage sheer, as you don't want anything to shine through your foundation. For the best results, paint on with a fine-tipped brush or smooth on to the skin with the fingertips — the heat generated in this way will help blend the product into the skin. Leave to settle for a few minutes before blotting with a tissue to absorb any excess oil, then apply foundation as usual.

3

six secrets for a flawless complexion

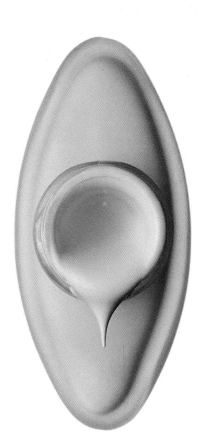

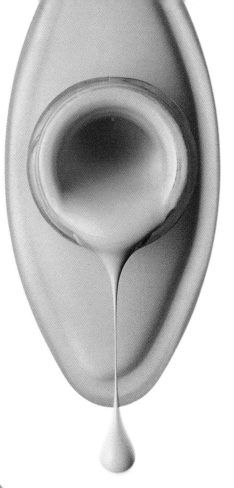

TRADE SECRETS

If you have dark circles under your eyes, mix concealer with a hint of peach or yellow colour corrector. To brighten sallow skin, add a little lilac base to your foundation. Use colour correctors sparingly and blend thoroughly so that they go undetected. Be wary of using white around the eyes, to avoid looking like a panda. If you have networks of blue veins on the eyelids, your foundation or concealer should be sufficient to mask these out.

4

MASTER MIX

To make application foolproof, try mixing a small amount of the colour corrector with a liquid foundation. Blend on the back of the hand and then dab on where needed before using your usual foundation over the rest of your face. Many foundations are too pink for the skin, but these can be custom-blended to create the perfect colour match by mixing with a yellow colour corrector.

5

6

POWDER OPTIONS

Steer clear of colour-correcting face powders. By the time you have used the primer and smoothed on your foundation, you shouldn't need to use them. Unless you really know what you're doing, they will cast an unsightly hue on the skin which tells everyone that you've been dabbling with colour correctors. The only exception is yellow-toned powder, which can be dusted over the skin to create a flattering finish or mixed with your existing powder, especially if that looks too pink on the skin.

CORRECTIONWORK

SHADOW FIX
If your choice of eyeshadow looks wrong, you can lift off the colour without disrupting the rest of your eye make-up: dip a clean cotton bud in foundation and then gently roll it over eyeshadow. This will remove the eyeshadow without disturbing your mascara and eyeliner. Alternatively, sweep a damp make-up sponge over the eyelid to tone the colour down.

CREASE WEAR
Creamy eyeshadows are renowned for creasing after several hours' wear. To overcome this, use an oil-free foundation as a pre-make-up base on the eyelids. Some make-up artists advise setting cream eyeshadows with a dusting of translucent powder to help them stay put. Alternatively, just smooth your fingertips over your eyelids every few hours

POWDER COLLECTION
If tiny particles of eyeshadow tend to collect under your eyes during application, deal with the problem by dipping a large brush in loose face powder and patting it under the eyes first. Stray particles of eyeshadow will collect here and then, when you've finished, the powder can be removed with a large make-up brush in one go.

BLUSH STROKES
If you add the finishing touches to your make-up by dusting on blusher only to find it looks too intense, use a foundation sponge and lightly press over the cheek area to lift off some of the product. Using your fingertips, gently rub your cheeks to blend in any existing make-up that is still there, then set with a light dusting of face powder.

follow quick-fix solutions to rectify mistakes

UNEVEN LINES

If, after applying, you find your pencil or liquid eyeliner is not straight or the line is of uneven thickness, you can always use the tip of a cotton bud to smudge the line so the effect looks intentional. As a foolproof way to ease application, steady the hand brushing on the eyeliner on a hard surface and look down into a mirror you've left resting there.

LIFT OFF

Overly made-up brows will not create a very flattering finish. If you realize you have been too heavy-handed with your pencil while defining, make your brows look more natural by running a cotton bud over the top to lift off some of the colour. Then wipe your index finger over them, brushing the hairs in the opposite direction to their natural growth, and finish off by reshaping.

LIGHTEN UP

Dark lipsticks do not suit everyone. If you have applied your lip colour and found it is too dark or does not go with your total make-up look, tone down the colour by coating the lips with gloss and then blotting the colour away using a tissue. Alternatively, massage a small amount of beige or gold lipstick on to the lips as a top coat to lighten the colour.

TWO TONE

If your foundation is not suited to your skin colour, you could end up looking like a mismatched beauty. To prevent this, never test-run new foundation shades on the back of your hand, as the tone of the skin here will differ from that of your face. Instead, always try out new shades over the jawline and the neck to get a natural-looking transition between face and neck.

BEAUTY INTELLIGENCE

1 To create an illusion of greater lash length, plant a mascara wand at the base of your lashes and gently roll it horizontally as you glide it through the lashes.

2 Always be careful when you are applying mascara to your lower eyelashes, remembering that if you have small eyes this can easily make them look distorted.

3 For the best results, opt for lip and cheek colours which are of a similar depth to your choice of eyeshadow, to ensure that the overall look is not unbalanced.

4 If you have thin lips, always choose pale shades of lipstick as these make lips look much fuller, while dark and intense colours make lips look smaller.

5 A clever play on colour can make the lips look soft and yet dramatic at the same time. Blend different shades of one colour for an interesting finish.

If you're running late and don't have time to define your brows, slick them down with a small amount of moisturizer, which will keep any unruly hairs in place.

6

7

Once you have applied your lipstick, you can go on to seal in the colour and simultaneously protect your lips by painting over a fine top coat of vitamin E oil.

You should always apply eye gel under your eyeshadow to act as the perfect fixative for make-up. It will also serve to condition the delicate skin around your eyes.

8

9

If lipstick tends to end up on your teeth after applying, put your index finger in your month, pout and then withdraw it. This will usually sort out the problem.

To improve the staying power of foundation, after application blot the skin with a tissue to remove any excess oil in the product, as this might spoil your overall look.

10

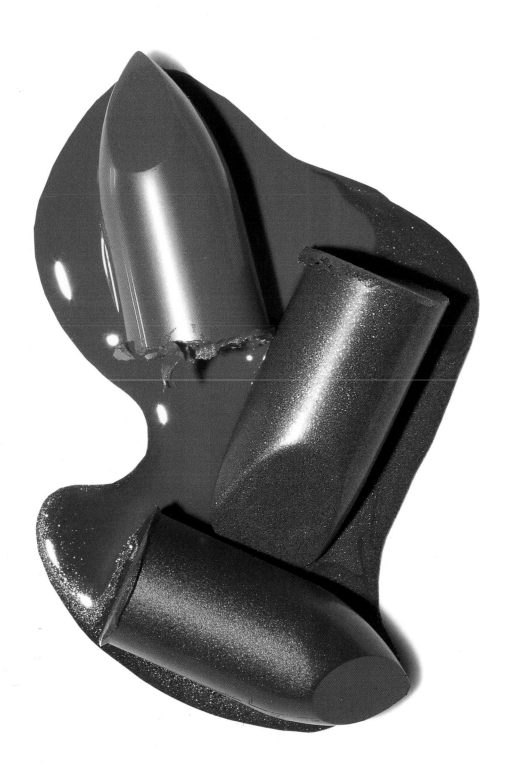

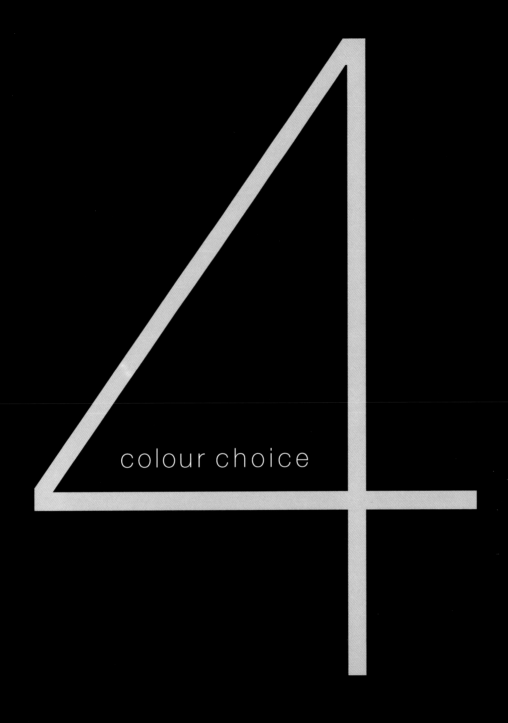

colour choice

Colour says a lot about your personality and mood. For example, wearing red shows that you are outgoing; pink suggests femininity; green reflects sincerity and balance; and violet means that you are artistic. Choose your colours according to your mood, but also look out for shades that harmonize with your natural colouring and your skin tone.

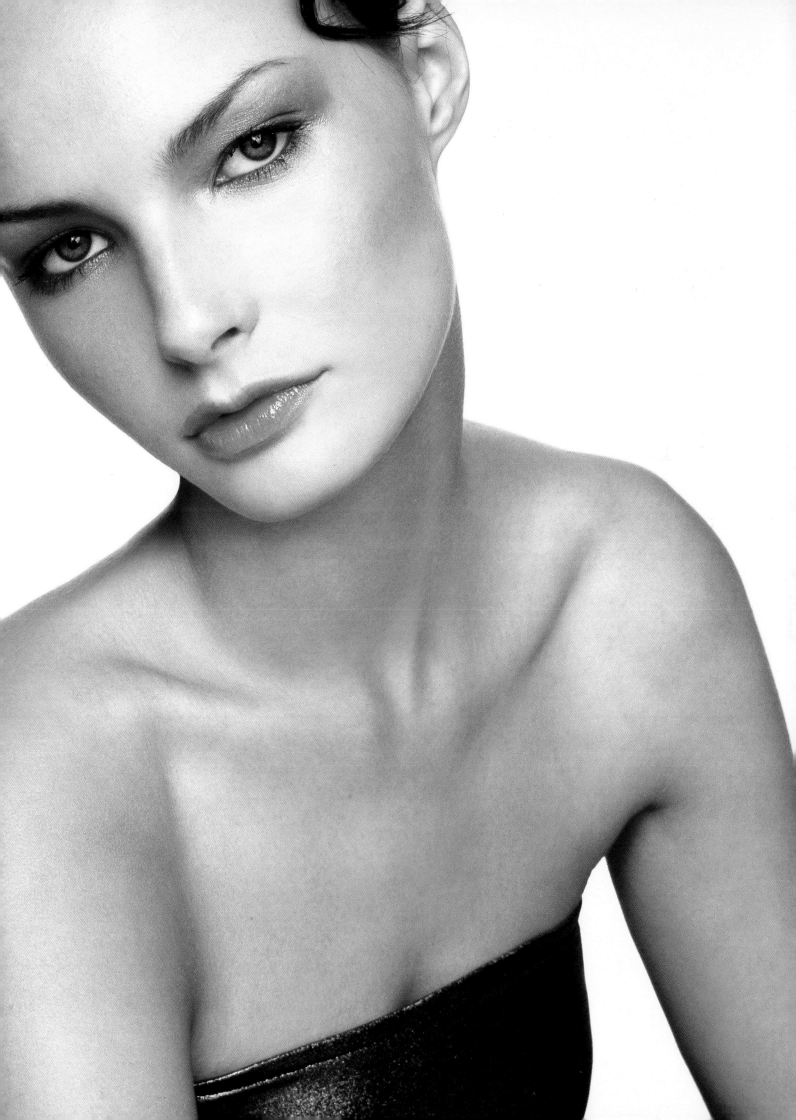

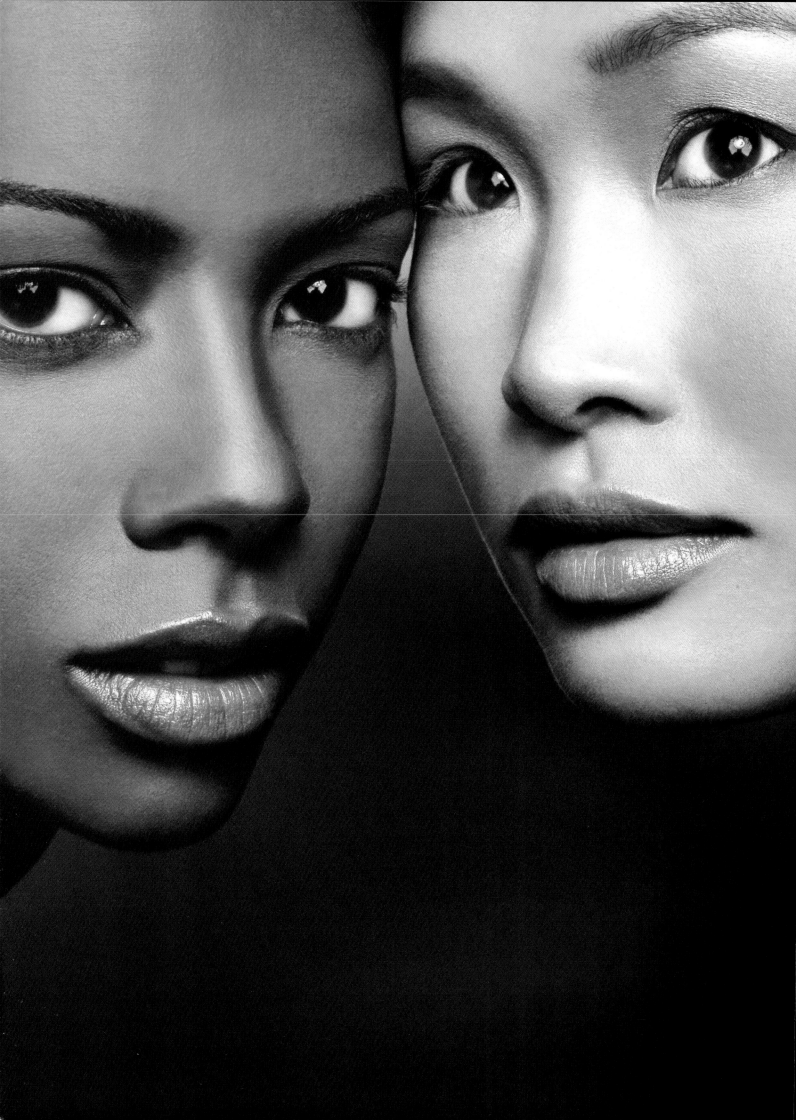

FAIR SKIN

Don't be tempted to use foundation in a shade darker than your natural skin tone to give more colour. Go for one with a subtle yellow undertone to warm the skin, and avoid pink-based shades, which can look ruddy. Choose an apricot blusher for a warm glow. For the eyes, navy blue, terracotta pink, silver and olive will suit you, while russet, gold, caramel, brown pink and electric blue will not. Find a lipstick that works without any other make-up. This colour will make your skin, hair and eyes look their best. Try nude, rosy brown and beige pink, and avoid cool tones, which can make you look drawn.

MEDIUM-TONED SKIN

This is the most common skin tone among Caucasian women and should be primed with a foundation that has a yellow undertone to warm the complexion. Avoid foundation colours that are too pale, as they can make you look washed out, but equally, if your foundation is too dark, it can make your skin look dirty, so choose carefully. For cheeks you should be looking at muted tawny and rose shades, avoiding anything with a strong orange base. Go for beige, slate, moss, bronze and mushroom eyeshadows, staying away from all the jewel colours, and from fuchsia pink, silver, pale blue and black.

OLIVE SKIN

Mediterranean skins look best with warmer tones of make-up. Avoid brown on the face, as it can look lifeless. Be wary of pink- or orange-toned foundation, as it looks mask-like. Opt for yellow-based shades that are not too dark. For the cheeks, warm pink shades look good; avoid stark contrasts of red or orange. Gold or bronze highlighters are flattering. For the eyes, choose browns mixed with terracotta and purples, midnight blue, rosy pink, browns and greens. Avoid pearly whites, greys, taupes and dusty browns, which will look ashy. For natural lip colours, go for rosy beige, deep reds and sheer browns.

DARK SKIN

Skin tone can vary across the face, so invest in two or three shades of base to balance the complexion. Generally, very dark skin needs foundation with a slight blue undertone, medium skin a red-yellow and light skin a soft gold. If you can't find the exact colour you want, try mixing shades. For cheek definition, apricot, dusky pink, rose and bronze enhance light skin; deep plum, currant and dark rose suit medium skin; and dark skin usually looks best with no blusher. For the lips, red, burgundy, blackberry, peach, purple and caramel will all work well, and can also be used to disguise uneven pigmentation.

ORIENTAL SKIN

Oriental women tend to have smooth, poreless caramel skin, so should use yellow-toned foundation and powder, avoiding powder that's translucent, as it can make the skin look washed out, and dulls natural warmth. To give the cheeks definition, medium and deep skin tones will suit tawny or rose shades of blusher (avoid bright pink and orange shades – they're too hard and garish) and pale skins will look good in soft pinks. For the lips, look for shades of clove, raisin or red-brown, and plum with undertones of brown, red or mauve. Avoid orange-red and light brown shades, which make the skin look muddy.

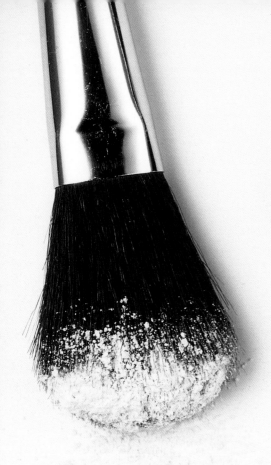
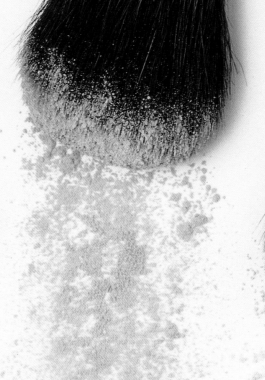

1

BLUE

Blue is no more or less wearable than any other colour. Choose from the deepest sea blue to the range of sheer pastels which create petrol-slick finishes. Deeper shades will suit mature women, while the softer, pale colours look better on younger skins. When experimenting with shades of blue, don't be put off by colours in their palettes, where they will look much more intense than they really are. To incorporate a hint of blue into your eye make-up, why not try defining the eyes with a blue kohl pencil, eyeliner or mascara?

2

PURPLE

Choose from the palest shade of lavender, heather or violet to shade the eyes, and use richer, stronger shades of blackberry, deep plum and vermilion to colour the lips. If you're wearing purple on the eyes, make-up artists advise using just one colour over the lid and defining the lash line with the same shade in a deeper tone. To balance the face, use colours for the lips and cheeks that are of a similar depth to the eyes, so the overall look is not too strong. Create an interesting lipstick finish by applying a layer of gold under deep vermilion.

3

PINK

Pink will suit most skin tones if you pick the right shade. The colour is very flattering to younger skins and can be used as a wash of colour on the cheeks, lips and eyes. You should avoid wearing pinks if your skin has a tendency to look red, as they will only accentuate the fact. For perfect pink eyes, make-up artists advise sticking to sheer textures, since they will illuminate rather than cover the eyes.

six secrets for wearing colour successfully

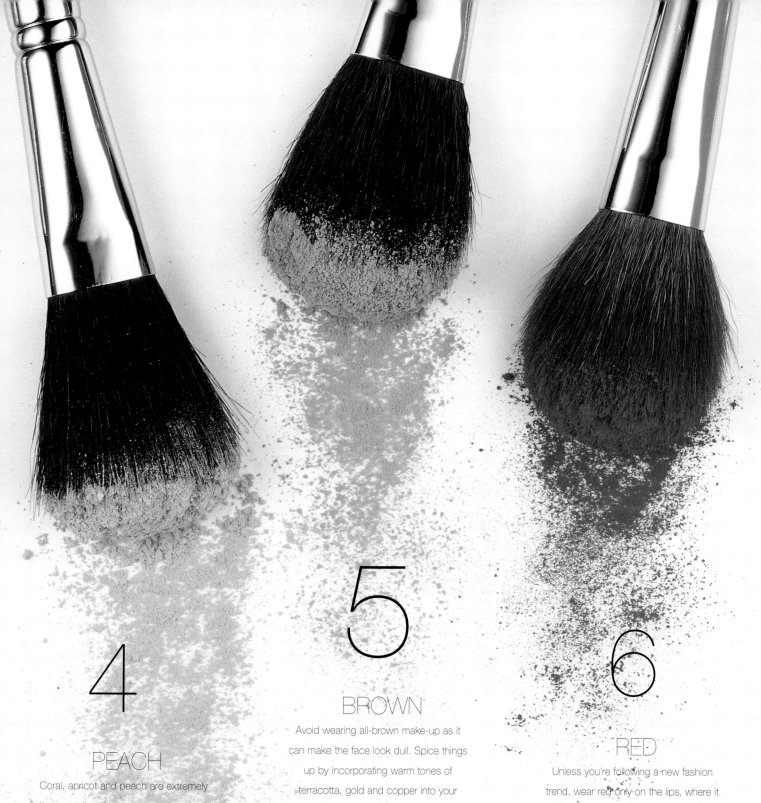

4

PEACH

Coral, apricot and peach are extremely flattering on the skin as long as they have a yellow undertone. They are a new way of creating natural-looking make-up, especially if you are stuck in a rut and always wear brown. Look for pale rather than gaudy shades. Do not match lips, nails and cheeks by defining with the same colour; look instead for different depths of the same shade to create a more flattering effect. Avoid flat, opaque finishes and go for glossy, shimmering textures that impart luminosity to the skin.

5

BROWN

Avoid wearing all-brown make-up as it can make the face look dull. Spice things up by incorporating warm tones of terracotta, gold and copper into your palette, and go for a combination of different textures and finishes to give features definition. If you have medium-toned skin, don't wear shades of brown that are too pale, as they can leave you looking washed out.

6

RED

Unless you're following a new fashion trend, wear red only on the lips, where it can make a strong beauty statement, especially if you have pale skin and dark hair. When selecting a lipstick, avoid cool or bluish reds if you have red, brown or black hair, as they can look dated. Blondes will suit any shade of red, but olive skins should opt for brown-based or wine and blackberry shades, while black skins should choose mahogany. For a soft approach, use a sheer red lipstick to add a hint of colour.

TEXTURE TWIST

Make-up is now available in every conceivable texture to give the skin a range of flattering finishes. The secret is to perfect your method of application: if you opt for total shine, you could end up looking a little greasy unless you are a professional; on the other hand, matt make-up can leave your face looking flat and lifeless. For the best results, aim for the middle ground and attempt a combination of matt and shimmering make-up on the face. Try teaming glistening skin with matt lips and frosted eyes, or a matt complexion with metallic-shaded eyes and glossy lips.

SHINING TRUE

The new generation of shimmery make-up gives a soft, petrol-slick finish that captures the light in a flattering way. You can choose from iridescent face and body powders, pearlized blushers, an array of metallic eyeshadows, lip tints and shimmery nail colours. Skin should glow without looking sparkly. There is a crucial difference between gleam and glitter. To give your skin a glistening finish, you can mix a shimmering fluid with your foundation before smoothing it on. To achieve a natural look, apply shimmer to the areas of the face which naturally catch the light, such as the tops of cheekbones. If you have very oily skin, do not try to achieve a glistening finish or you could end up with an oil-slick on your face. Instead use an oil-free foundation which dries to a matt finish. A foolproof way to apply shimmer is to dust on a pearlized powder, slick on lip gloss or use an iridescent cream eyeshadow on the eyelid. To break up shimmer on the face, you can use a matt kohl pencil to add definition to frosted eyes or team iridescent eyes and lips with a matt blusher. For a subtle finish, experiment with pearlized eyeliners. These can give the eyes a flattering finish if a light shade, like a silver or soft blue, is applied on the inner corners of the upper and lower lashes and blended out to fade gradually. When looking for lipsticks, you should opt for a shimmery finish which contains fewer reflective pigments and is much more flattering than any of its frosted counterparts, which have more pigments and are much drier.

MATT MAKE-OVER

Matt make-up is the perfect accompaniment to offset high shine. Every make-up kit should contain matt eyeshadow, which will come into its own for shading and contouring the eyes; matt pencils will add definition to frosted eyes; and a matt blusher, which will work in harmony with a shimmery highlighter. To really get to grips with wearing all-matt make-up, you will need to steer clear of foundation, powder, blusher, eyeshadow and lipstick, since they dry to a matt finish and so will make the face look flat and lifeless. Matt lipsticks look great but are reputed to have a drying effect on the lips; also, as they wear off, they can leave a rather unsightly stain on the lips. One simple way of geting round these problems is to always choose 'semi-matt' formulations.

TEXTURE TRANSFORMATION

There are several simple steps you can follow to either transform matt products into shimmering finishes or conversely turn high-shine products into matt formulations. One of the easiest ways to convert any matt product, whether it is lipstick or eyeshadow, into a glossy finish is to slick it with Vaseline or lip gloss. If you want to create a more subtle shimmer, simply sweep a wash of pearlized ivory highlighter over eyeshadow, blusher or lipstick. To tone down high-shine lipstick, press face powder on to the lips using a velour powder puff or blot the lips with a tissue to remove the glossy finish and leave a stain of colour on the lips.

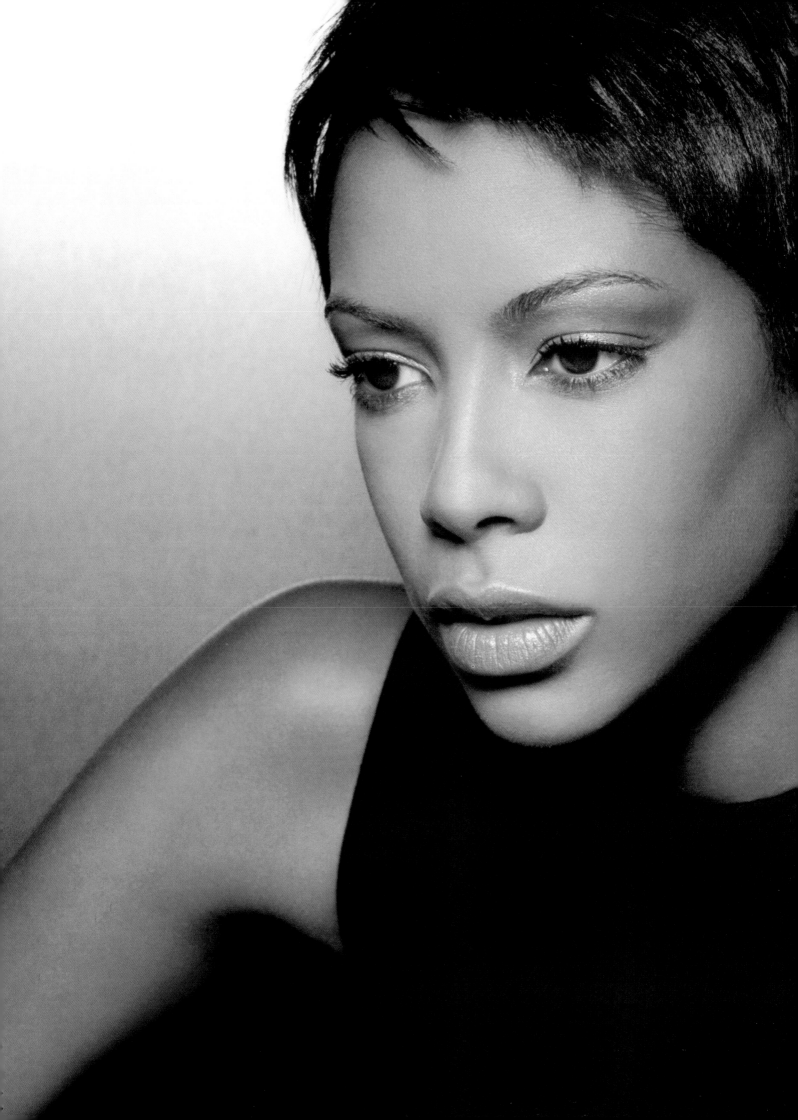

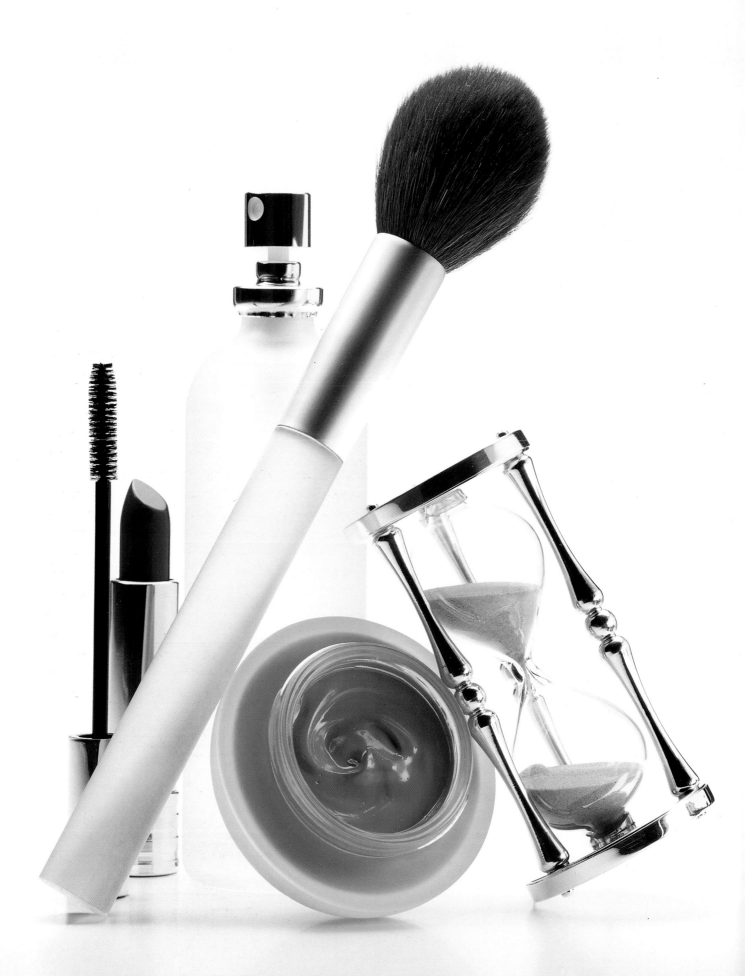

MATURE FACES

FOUNDATION As we age, our skin changes, becoming much drier and more prone to flushing. The tone is less vibrant, fine lines and wrinkles are more apparent, and the lips loose their fullness. Look for cosmetics that will work in harmony with your skin's condition and colour. Play up your strong features and use cosmetics to draw attention away from fine lines and wrinkles. Drier skins will benefit from oil-based foundations. Look for creamy formulations that will glide on smoothly, so that you avoid dragging the skin. Always wear moisturizer as an undercoat, to plump up the skin cells, and look for a formula that contains a sunscreen to help prevent more age and sun spots developing on the face. Concealer is one of the mature woman's greatest allies. It can be used in order to tone down flushed skin, to disguise broken capillaries, to mask changes in pigmentation and to minimize deep shadows. Stick concealers are preferable to creamy preparations which are applied with wands. You should always opt for yellow-toned concealers to complement your skin tone. Ruddy-looking complexions can be evened out with colour-correcting bases (see page 64).

BLUSHER Cheeks which are prone to flushing and have broken capillaries should be defined with soft browns and peaches, rather than pinks, to avoid accentuating redness. Wearing blusher helps to draw attention away from crow's-feet around the eyes. Creamy formulations can give mature skins a flattering finish. Make-up artists suggest that you avoid using face powder later in life, as it can emphasize fine lines and wrinkles. If, however, you want to use powder, choose pressed rather than loose, as it is easier to control during application.

EYES Be very wary of using bright colours or tricky colour combinations, as they can make the eyes appear smaller and more deep-set than they really are. The aim is to contour the eyes without letting colour creep into any fine lines around them. Look for warm browns, taupes, olives, lavender and chestnut red to shade the eyes. Avoid dark eye colours – certain shades of dark grey can make the eyelids look very heavy, especially if you are prone to tired or sallow-looking skin. Eyeshadow one shade darker than your foundation is a great option for day wear. If you feel that your eyes are more 'droopy' than they used to be, do not coat the eyelid with colour but instead define the socket line and shade along the lower lash line to 'lift' them. Bear in mind that matt finishes are more flattering than pearlized, frosted products as you get older. Make sure you steer clear of bright white frosted highlighters and shimmering shadows, and look for powdery eyeshadows as opposed to cream or gel formulations, as they will stay where they are supposed to be and not crease into fine lines and wrinkles. Define sparse brows by applying eye pencil in small, feathered strokes rather than one line, which will look very unnatural. Coat the eyelashes with a lash-building mascara.

LIPS If you want to draw attention away from your eyes, use a strong colour of lipstick. But remember that very dark tones can look hard and make small lips appear mean and surly. If you do opt for a brighter lip colour, take steps before application to prevent it feathering into fine lines around the mouth: coat the lips with a lip liner (it contains waxes and less oil, which makes it stay put longer than lipstick), blot with powder and then smooth on your lipstick, blot with a tissue and reapply lipstick.

NOCTURNAL BEAUTY

PREP WORK If you want your daytime look to take you right through to the early hours of the morning, follow these few simple steps. Slip a cleansing wipe into your bag, ready to be used at the end of the day to freshen up the complexion and to remove what is left of your daytime make-up. Do not use it on the eyes or on the sensitive areas around the eyes; instead you should wipe over with a damp cotton-wool pad or with the tip of a moistened cotton bud to clean up. Smooth a damp tissue over the complexion and then gently press moisturizer or a special skin-boosting preparation into the skin.

MAKE-UP BASE For a flawless evening base, apply two layers of foundation. Leave the first, which should be very light, to dry, then follow with a second layer. This way, no matter how late you stay out, your foundation will last. At night artificial light will be harsh and can accentuate shadows around the eyes, so you'll need your concealer. Candlelight, however, will be kinder, casting a flattering halo of yellow light on the skin.

EVENING GLAMOUR Beauty after dark is not about wearing lots of make-up in an abundance of different colours. Always aim to look sophisticated in an understated way. Neutral day-wear tones tend to disappear at night, so if you don't feel comfortable with the idea of drastically altering your make-up looks, simply opt for the colours that you normally wear but choose slightly darker shades. In this way, you will create a more dramatic effect but one that is not too far removed from your daytime appearance. Alternatively, incorporate metallic, not glittery, finishes into your existing make-up palette. Blend gold with brown and copper, and silver with blue, pink and cherry red.

NIGHT-TIME DRAMA For a modern look, make either the eyes or the lips the focal point of beauty. If you try to accentuate both features, the results can look dated and sometimes too harsh and artificial. If you choose to strengthen the eyes, use a wash of colour on the lips. Alternatively, paint on a strong shade of lipstick and simply run liner along the upper lashes, adding a couple of coats of mascara to the lashes.

SKIN LUMINOSITY Bare skin that is on show in cutaway clothing should be given a radiant finish. Smooth on moisturizer and then dust with a shimmery face powder or bronzing powder. For a golden glow, prime the skin with self-tan a couple of days prior to your evening out. For the best results, smooth on to freshly exfoliated skin. The secret to no-streak tans is to blend thoroughly. If you normally spend five minutes applying body moisturizer, take double the time with self-tan – it will be well worth it. Always wash your hands afterwards. Avoid washing the body with alkaline soaps, as they can alter the colour, and do not have a bath or shower after applying self-tan, as it will interfere with the colour process. Do not forget the earlobes and the upper side of the hands – the bits people do tend to forget – as these will give your game away. If you end up with streaks of colour, gently exfoliate the area or smooth on whitening toothpaste, leave for five minutes and then remove.

FRAGRANT FINISH Perfume is a must for the evening. Don't think of dabbing it on behind the ears – the numerous oil glands located here can alter the balance of your perfume's ingredients. Instead dab it on to the pulse points on the inside of the wrists, your cleavage or the nape of your neck.

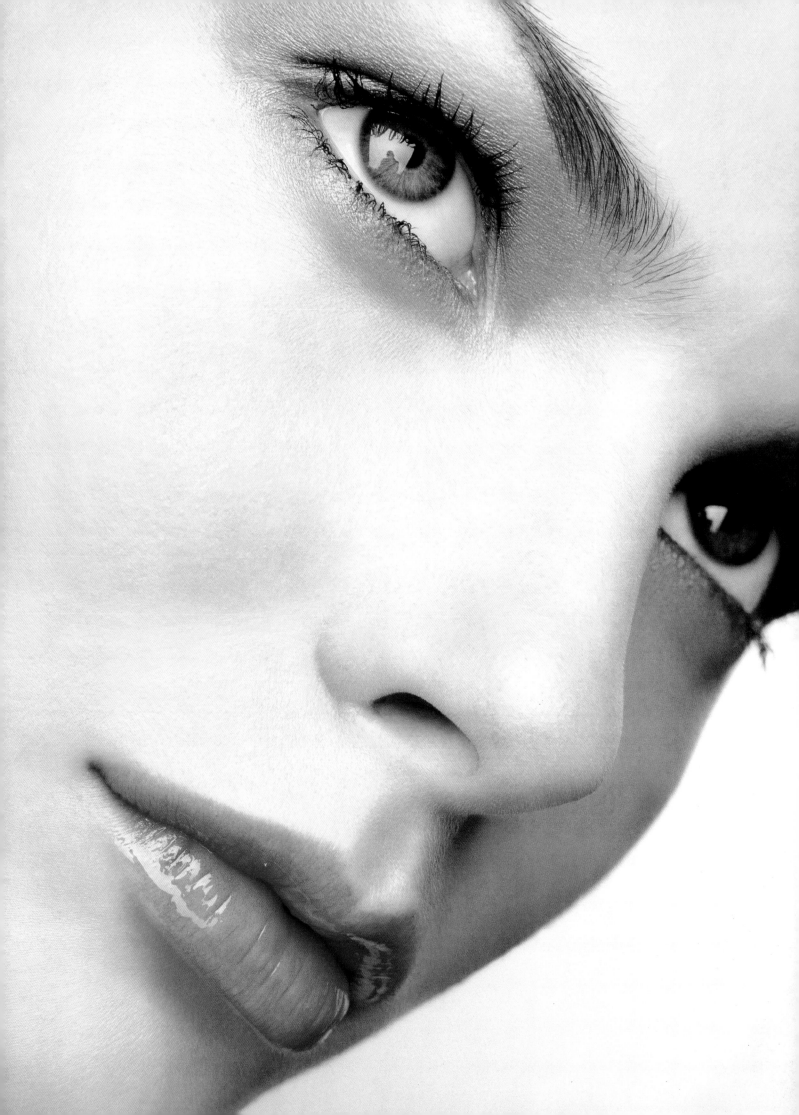

STAYINGPOWER

LASTING BLUSH

Dusting on powder blusher takes a couple of seconds but it can disappear within hours of application. To improve its staying power, make-up artists recommend this foolproof tip: smooth on a cream blusher and then dust with a powder formula in a similar shade. The powder blusher will act as a setting agent over the creamy formula for lasting wear.

NAIL WORK

To make nail polish more durable, always apply a base coat before painting the nails with polish. This will create a tacky finish on the nail surface, even when dry, which then acts as an adhesive base for the polish. Also, by wearing a base coat you will help to strengthen the nails and will prevent more brightly coloured polishes staining the nail plate.

LIP COAT

Some make-up artists use a non-toxic, water-based felt-tip pen to stain the lips as a base coat. This is one way to guarantee that lip colour remains true, and is great for creating a 'bee-stung' look on the lips. To remove, simply massage your normal creamy cleanser into the lips, leave on for a few seconds to break down the colour and then wipe off with cotton wool.

SHADOW BOOST

You can always extend the staying power of your eyeshadow by smoothing on an oil-free foundation to the eyelids as a base before applying eye colour. Oil-free formulations tend to glide on and not slide off, whereas their oil-based equivalents are not so long-lasting and therefore cannot provide a good adhesive base for eye make-up.

follow these steps to prolong the life of your make-up

LIPSTICK FIX

You can invest in long-wear lipsticks, but some are drying on the lips and require special removers. Instead, use a lipliner in a shade close to your natural lip colour, shade the entire lip area and then coat with lipstick. Blot gently with a tissue and reapply lip colour, then repeat the process until a stain of colour remains on the lips. Finally, add your last coat of lipstick.

LASH POWER

You can improve the staying power of mascara by dusting your eyelashes with a little face powder before coating them with mascara. This will also make the lashes appear much fuller and more voluptuous. If your mascara does not normally stay put, avoid wearing on the lower lashes and find a long-lasting formulation, as these are designed to be more durable.

BASE CONTROL

To improve the longevity of foundation, after applying a liquid formula blot the face with a tissue. This will remove any excess surface oil which might interfere with the product's staying power. For maximum coverage, you can always add another thin layer of foundation and then finish off the look by setting this with a light dusting of face powder.

LASTING LINER

To make liquid or pencil eyeliner stay in place longer, after applying trace the line with a fine brush dipped in powder eyeshadow or translucent face powder. The powder will literally set the eyeliner. Alternatively, you could choose a waterproof formulation. These are more durable and contain special ingredients that are designed to withstand heat and humidity.

BEAUTY INTELLIGENCE

1 For a fresh, dewy complexion, you need to avoid powder overload, so apply it only to those areas prone to shine, like your nose, chin and forehead.

2 Make eyeliner application easier by lifting your eyelid at the eyebrow with one finger, so the skin is taut, and try applying the liner in one smooth stroke.

3 If you want to use blusher to give cheeks that sculpted look, suck them in and softly contour the upper shape, taking care not to create streaks of colour.

4 In order to make your eyes appear larger, make-up artists recommend that you leave a fine line between the edge of your eyelashes and the eyeliner.

5 As you get older, avoid metallic eyeshadows – glistening textures will only highlight fine lines and wrinkles. You will find that matt finishes are much more flattering.

When selecting shades of eyeshadow, always take into account the size of your eyes. If you have small eyes, dark colours can make them smaller.

6

7

To give your pout definition, shade the outer corners of the lips with a pencil darker than your lipstick and dab lip gloss on to the centre of the lower lip.

If you want to play down the size of your lips, do not define the outer shape with a lip liner, as this will accentuate the fullness, and always wear a pale colour.

8

9

If your complexion looks tired and lifeless, avoid foundation, which will only make things worse, and get to work with a concealer and tinted moisturizer.

If your skin is prone to clogged pores, you will need to look for a foundation that does not contain mineral oil, which is more than likely to aggravate the condition.

10

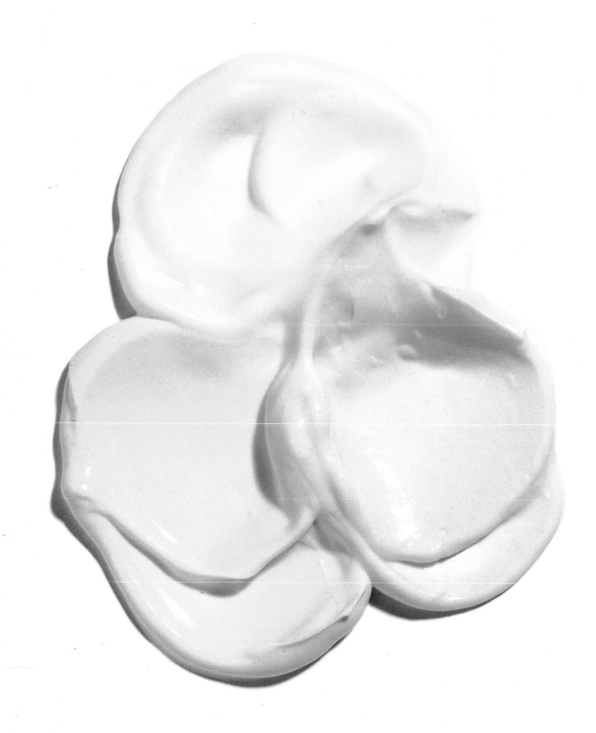

beauty upkeep

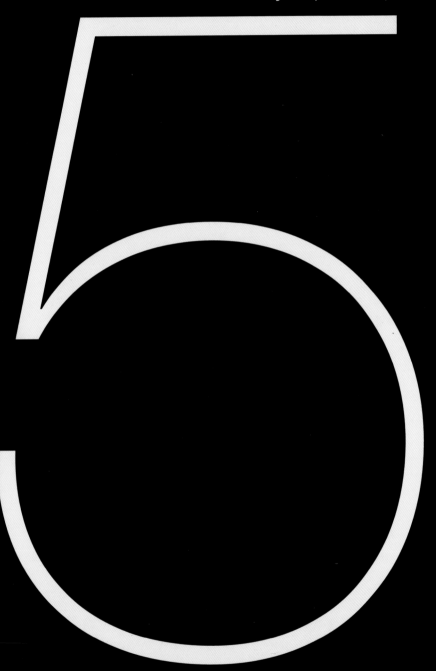

Good grooming might seem effortless, but there's a fine art to getting everything just right. It is not about sporting the most fashionable eye colour or the latest nail length. The secret is to have radiant skin, groomed brows and polished nails. If you take the following simple steps to attend to your beauty needs, you will be well on your way to looking good.

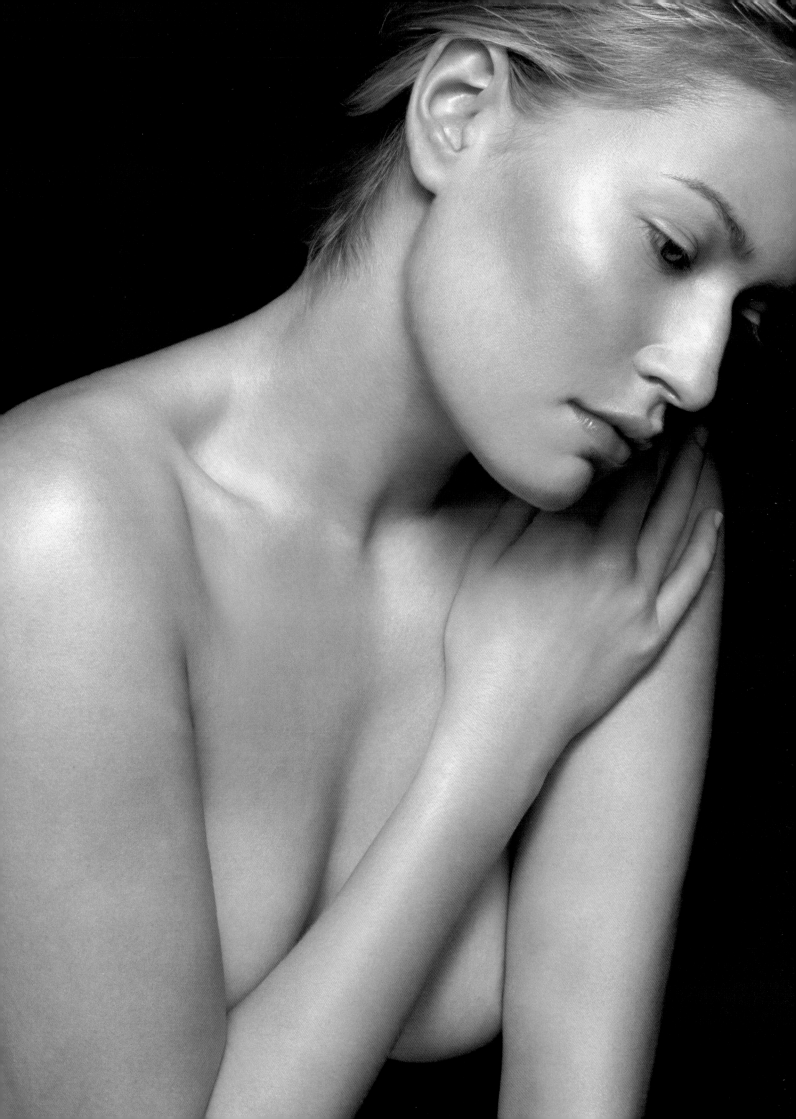

SKIN-CARE
ESSENTIALS

EXFOLIATOR

should be used at least once a week to buff
away dead skin and improve circulation.
If you have delicate, sensitive skin, look
for a formulation which contains special
ingredients that literally dissolve dead skin,
avoiding ones with granules, as they
can be rather abrasive.

REFRESHERS

such as floral waters are not a necessity but
they can be used to wipe over the face
after cleansing or sprayed on as an instant
pick-me-up. Avoid alcohol-based toners,
which can strip the skin of essential
moisture, causing dryness.

WASH-OFF
CLEANSER

or a pH-balanced cleansing bar is
ideal for use in the bath or shower every
morning. In combination with a facial
cleansing brush, you can exfoliate and
cleanse your face in one go.

EYE MAKE-UP
REMOVER

is essential for cleansing the delicate area
around the eyes. Normal cleansers should
not be used here as they can contain
fragrance and other ingredients which might
irritate the eyes. Look for non-oily formulas
and work gently from the outer corner
of the eye inwards, taking care not
to drag the skin.

FACE MASKS

are a must if you want radiant skin. Once a week oily skins will benefit from a deep-cleansing face mask enriched with clay to help shift impurities and unclog the pores. Dry skins need a creamy hydrating formula; stressed skins need a soothing mask which doesn't contain potential irritants; and normal skins need a gentle cleansing formula to remove dead skin and those by-products of modern living: pollution and smoke.

CREAM CLEANSER

or oil-based variants, will make light work of shifting make-up and impurities, and is ideal for use at night. Massage into the skin in small circular motions, and leave for a few seconds to dissolve impurities. Remove with damp cotton wool or moistened sponges.

MOISTURIZER

used daily, is essential for all skin types. Look for a formulation containing a sunscreen, as well as antioxidants to prevent premature ageing and sufficient hydration to suit your skin.

NIGHT CREAMS

are a good investment as the skin's recuperative power is at its height from 11 p.m. to 1 a.m. and they contain special ingredients that will help.

EYE CREAM

can help protect delicate skin around the eyes. For day wear, choose a formula enriched with UV protectors and antioxidants. Gently pat into the skin under the eyes and along the orbital and brow bones. Heat from the skin will deliver the product where it's needed and if applied any closer, it might actually seep into the eyes and cause puffiness.

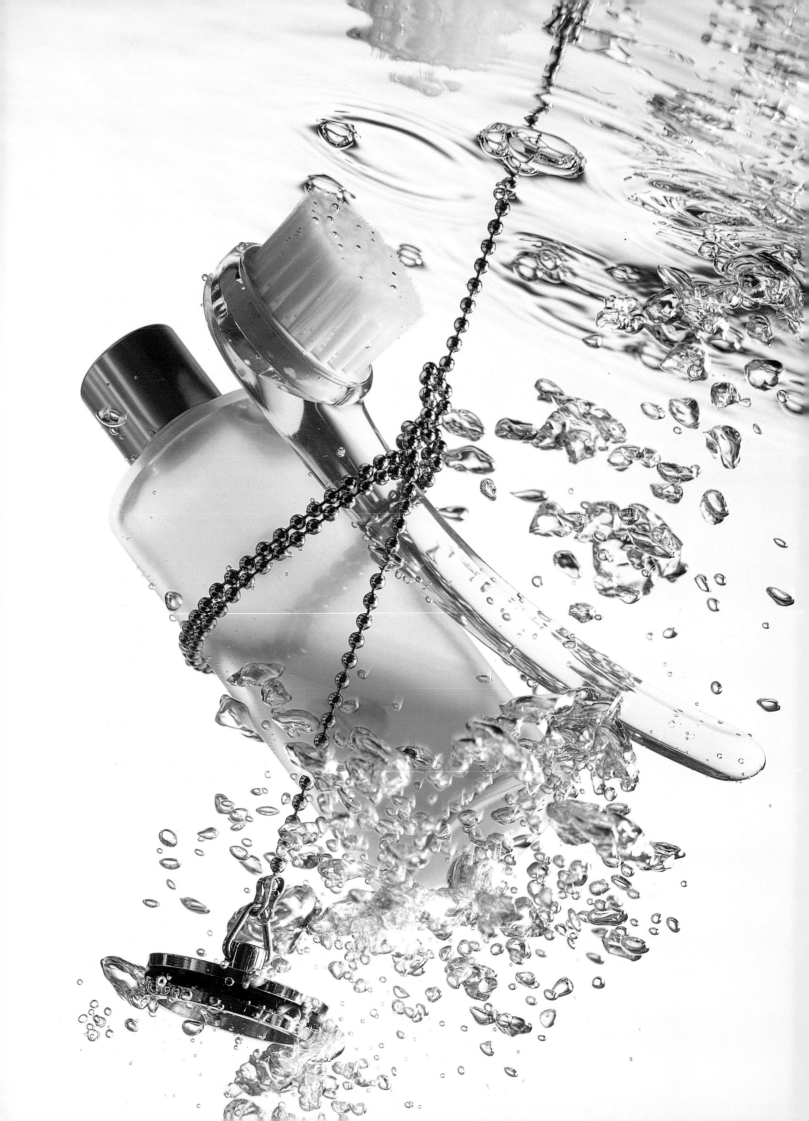

SKIN CARE

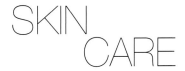

Whatever your particular skin type, there are three basic factors to bear in mind if you want a youthful-looking complexion. You will need to cleanse regularly, to hydrate properly and to provide protection from the elements before you address any of the problems that relate specifically to your type of skin. Your skin-care regime doesn't necessarily have to be time-consuming or entail the use of lots of different products.

CLEANSING
Don't over-cleanse the skin. Skin is meant to act as a barrier, keeping irritants out and moisture in. When you over-cleanse, you strip away essential lipids and cellular matter which are responsible for retaining the skin's moisture. This will lead to heightened sensitivity, which in turn can result in mild redness, rashes and dermatitis. Over-cleansing can also cause dehydration and premature ageing. The pores can become inflamed and irritated, upsetting the skin's cell-renewal process and leading to clogged pores and even to adult acne.

HYDRATING
Whether you opt for a gel, a cream or a lotion, you need to find a moisturizer that will suit your skin type. The skin can absorb only a finite number of ingredients and any over-rich or unsuitable products will simply clog the pores, leaving the way open for a variety of unsightly skin problems.

PROTECTING
The sun is the skin's deadliest enemy, being responsible for some 90 per cent of premature ageing. Always protect your skin with a product containing a sun protection factor of at least 15 – remember, even on the cloudiest days the sun's ultraviolet rays will penetrate the clouds. Those who want to look radiant and healthy should think about incorporating a self-tanning preparation into their beauty regime.

OILY SKINS
Look for products that control the activity of the sebaceous glands, as it is now possible to 'reprogram' this type of skin. Most sufferers fear that products containing oil will exacerbate the problem; though this isn't strictly true, it's best to opt for oil-free preparations. If you are prone to blackheads and clogged pores, steam your face over a bowl of near-boiling water, then slather on a deep-cleansing face mask once a week. This will literally vacuum-clean the skin. Don't try to avoid using moisturizer; otherwise you'll end up with dehydrated skin.

THIRSTY SKINS
These are either dry skins, which lack oil, or dehydrated skins, which lack water. Products exist to redress the balance. Dry skin is either hereditary or occurs as a result of harsh weather, exposure to the sun or age. Invest in a rich moisturizer, avoid wash-off cleansers and use creamy formulations. Do not use alcohol-based toners and fuel the skin internally with evening primrose oil. To treat dehydrated skin, exfoliate regularly, as a build-up of dead skin can stop products which draw atmospheric moisture in from working effectively.

SENSITIVE/STRESSED SKINS
These usually feel tight and look blotchy. They can flare up after trying new products, sun exposure and harsh weather. Avoid perfumed products or those with unnatural colorants, alcohol or chemical sunscreens. Creamy cleansers will be soothing. Shield delicate skins with products containing a suncreen and avoid those with alpha hydroxy acids (AHAs). Networks of broken blood vessels can occur on the nose and cheeks. Take preventive steps by using sunscreen and a rich protective barrier cream. Avoid exposure to extreme weather conditions, spicy foods and hot water.

COMBINATION SKINS
These are usually greasy in the T-zone, with all its sebaceous glands, and dry elsewhere. Most products now are formulated to work on surface dryness while controlling the underlying oiliness. Use a moisturizer which contains water and lipids, not oil; oil-free make-up; and wash-off cleansers. Avoid alcohol toners, instead choosing products with AHAs to decongest the skin and prevent clogged pores.

SKIN RADIANCE

PROFESSIONAL TOUCH Treat yourself to regular facials every six weeks and book in for a deep-cleansing facial twice a year. Avoid having facials during your period, as the skin is more prone to sensitivity then. After a facial, try not to wear make-up for at least two hours, to allow skin to breathe.

BACTERIA ALERT Every time you open a jar of face cream or a bottle of lotion and dip your fingers in, you are intruding bacteria, which can then affect the product's shelf life. Bottles with pump-dispensers offer a simple way of getting round this problem. Being air-tight, to stop the contents oxidizing on contact with the air, their design also means you can use the product without interfering with its ingredients.

SPOT ATTACK If you suffer from oily, problem skin you should avoid alcohol, caffeine, spices and foods containing iodides, like shellfish, as they can sometimes stimulate oil production. Some skin-care experts recommend leaving a dab of toothpaste on pimples overnight, so they dry out. Others suggest using eyedrops to take the redness out of them.

SOAP STRATEGY Some people swear that using soap and water is the secret to successful cleansing, but the experts tend not to recommend this approach. Conventional soaps often leave an alkaline residue on the skin which is hard to rinse off and can interfere with the efficiency of moisturizers. Always use a pH-balanced cleansing bar suited to your skin type and wet the skin with tepid water first. When rinsing your face, use only warm water, as water that is too hot can irritate the skin and have a drying effect. Over-cleansing oily skin will simply lead to an increase in oil production. In order to avoid drying oily skin out by over-cleansing, you should only cleanse at night.

STEAM-CLEANING Blackheads are caused by sebum blocking the hair follicles, not a build-up of dirt. Blackheads attain their colour when the sebum oxidizes on exposure to the air. If your skin is prone to blackheads and breakouts, it's advisable to steam your face every ten days. Boil a kettle and then pour boiling water into a large bowl. Leave to stand for thirty seconds, then put your face about 10cm above the bowl and cover your head with a towel so the steam does not escape and gets to work on your face. Stay like this for two to three minutes, then slather on a deep-cleansing face mask.

MASQUERADE To maintain skin radiance, incorporate a face mask into your weekly beauty regime. If your skin is oily, a deep-cleansing clay or mud mask, which literally vacuum-cleans the skin, will help. Dry skin will benefit from moisturizing masks with ingredients like hyaluronic acid, vegetable proteins, amino acids and essential fatty acids. Soothe temperamental skin with a mask containing anti-inflammatory ingredients such as camomile and sea algae. To boost normal or dull skin, look for an exfoliating mask that will buff away your dead skin cells.

CLEANLINESS You should always wash your hands before you touch your face and should avoid touching your skin unnecessarily. Clean the handset of your telephone regularly: beauty therapists suggest using an antibacterial wipe to remove the germs and bacteria that accumulate there, as these could cause irritation on the skin under the jaw and lead to breakouts.

WEATHER CHECK During the winter, if your skin is exposed to harsh weather conditions or you have to spend prolonged periods out of doors, you should smooth on an oil-based moisturizer. Don't use water-based moisturizers, which can literally freeze on the skin, disrupting its natural balance.

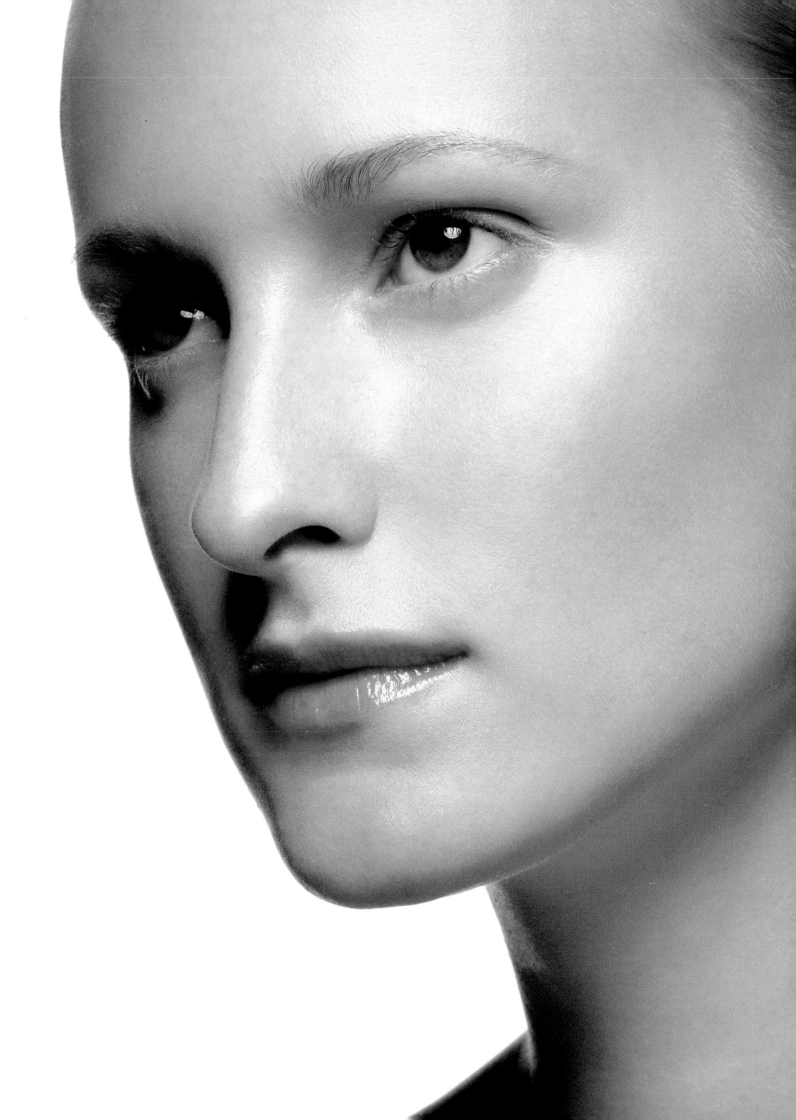

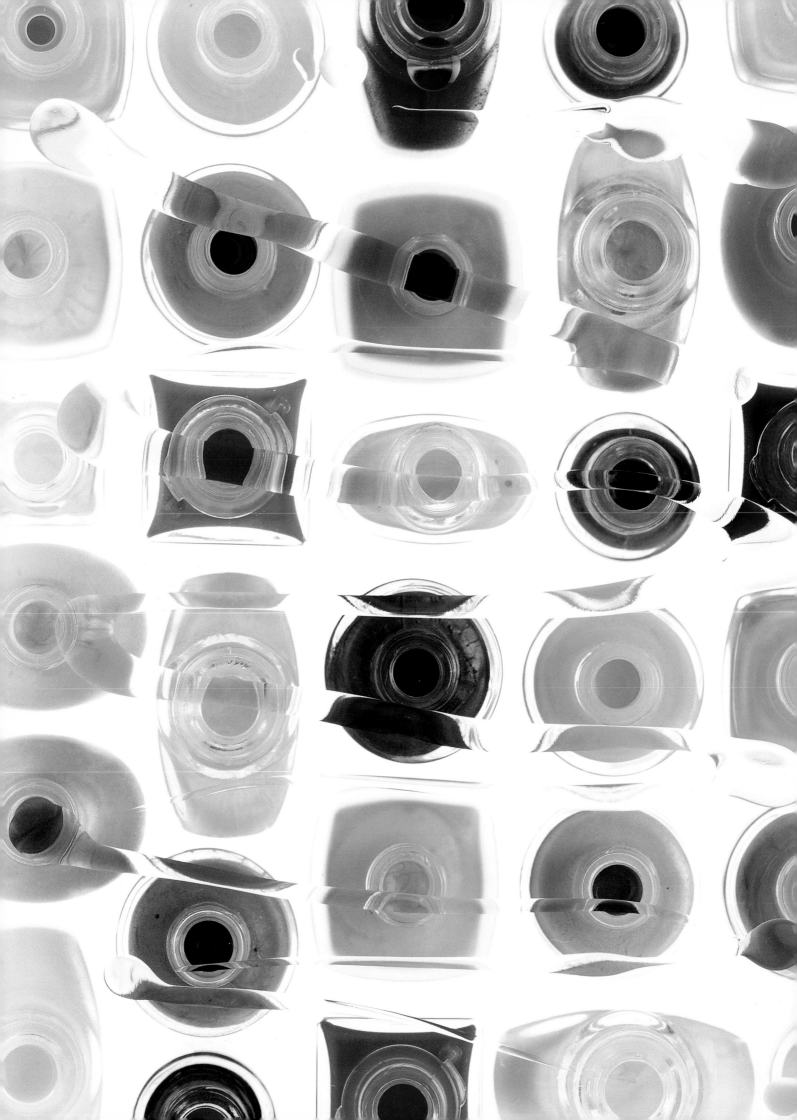

NAIL CARE

Diet plays an important part in nail condition. You should eat foods containing vitamins A, E and B complex, and the minerals calcium, zinc, magnesium and iodine. Contrary to popular belief, white spots on the nails don't necessarily mean a calcium deficiency. If only one or two nails are affected, they are more likely to be caused by external bruising. If you don't wear nail polish, run a buffer over the nails to boost their blood supply, which will promote growth and also enhance natural shine. But be gentle: over-zealous buffing can thin nails. It is also advisable to paint on hardener to protect your nails.

SHAPE UP

Manicurists recommend that you file your nails after a bath or shower, as the nails are more pliable then and so are less prone to flaking or breakages. Remember to work the file over the nails in one direction only; otherwise the heat you generate as you go back and forth will dry the nails out and also traumatize the nail plate. Short nails will always stay smart-looking for longer, whereas talons which extend way past the tips of the fingers are more susceptible to polish chips and breakages. You should leave the sides of the nails rounded and opt for square tips, as they will hold your polish better.

VARNISHING TRICKS

Before applying polish, always wash your hands with a non-lanolin soap to get rid of any residue from nail treatments, as these can weaken nail polish. Apply polish sparingly: the thinner each coat, the longer polish resists chipping. The first application should be almost transparent. If polish has set on the skin surrounding the nails, have a bath or shower and afterwards the polish will simply peel off. Never shake polish before application: this whips bubbles into the formula, which can cause chipping later on. Instead, simply turn the bottle upside-down and gently roll it between the palms of your hands.

DISAPPEARING ACT

Before removing nail polish, massage a drop of oil or moisturizer into the cuticles. This will prevent them drying out and stop the remover staining the polish into the nails. There is still great debate about whether you should use acetone-free or acetone nail polish remover. Acetone polish remover is the most effective to shift stubborn stay-put polishes but can cause nail dryness. To compensate, add a couple of drops of oil to the remover and shake well before using. If your nails become very dry, massage almond or jojoba oil into the nail plate morning and night to rehydrate and improve the condition.

COLOUR CODE

Sheer colours are the most user-friendly and make imperfections less noticeable. When buying pale polish, take your skin tone into account: opt for pink or clear if you have a pinkish skin tone; beige, peach or clear suits olive and yellow skin tones; while any shade suits black skin. When wearing bright or bold colours, use the skin on the inside of the wrist as a guide to see if cool or warm tones suit you. If your skin has a bluish tinge, polishes with cool undertones will work; if it has a yellow tone go for warm colours. As you get older avoid pale colours and natural shades since they can age the hands.

ONCE BITTEN

To put a stop to habitual nail-biting, have a professional manicure, then either paint on one of those harmless but foul-tasting colourless formulas to stop chewers or opt for a session with a hypnotherapist. Massage a drop of oil or cream into the cuticles and nails daily. If your nails start to look better, it will spur you on to stop biting for good. Once you've broken the habit, use a hardener to get the nails into optimum condition and treat yourself to regular manicures. As your nails start to grow and become healthy-looking, paint the tips with a white matt or pearlized polish. This will make them look longer.

CUTICLE CARE

It's best not to trim your cuticles. They are there to prevent bacteria getting in and causing infections, and unless you do it properly you'll be left with unsightly snags of skin around the nail. So, while you're in the bath or shower, gently push the nails back using a soft-bristled brush. This will attend to the cuticles, whisk away dead skin, pep up the circulation and smooth the nail surface. Cuticle creams enriched with alpha hydroxy acids are good for keeping cuticles in trim. Manicurists recommend applying daily, preferably before bathing or showering, so that the heat can increase absorption of the cream.

HANDY TIPS

If you suffer from dry hands and brittle nails, avoid using highly perfumed lotions because the alcohol in them may leave your skin feeling even drier and irritated. When you are outdoors, look for a handcream enriched with a sunscreen to prevent premature ageing. Preparations containing high doses of vitamin C will help prevent sun and age spots from developing. If these are already apparent on your hands, use a handcream that is enriched with hydroquinone to fade imperfections. Never apply handcream straight after painting your nails, because this can dull the surface of freshly polished nails.

NAIL STRENGTH

If your nails are weak, prone to split and break easily, step up the protein in your diet or try taking gelatin capsules. Some manicurists blame soft nails on a mineral deficiency or hypochlorhydrin (lack of stomach acid). This prevents the proper production of amino acids, which nails require to remain healthy and strong. Try taking a six-week course of nutritional supplements to eliminate hypochlorhydrin, but seek expert advice first. You could always paint on nail hardener with strengthening ingredients in the form of nylon fibres and resins. For maximum strength, keep your nails shortish and with square tips.

POLISH WORK

Once you have removed nail polish, if you are left with discoloured nails, drop two denture-cleansing tablets into quarter of a glass of water and use this solution with a nailbrush to gently scrub the nails. Help prolong the shelf life of your nail enamel by wiping the rim of an unsealed bottle with a little oil before replacing the lid. This will stop the lid sticking and will also ensure that the bottle is closed properly. If the bottle is not air-tight, the product will dry out and be unusable. Nail polish should always be stored in a cool place, as heat will expand the ingredients and can affect the product's consistency.

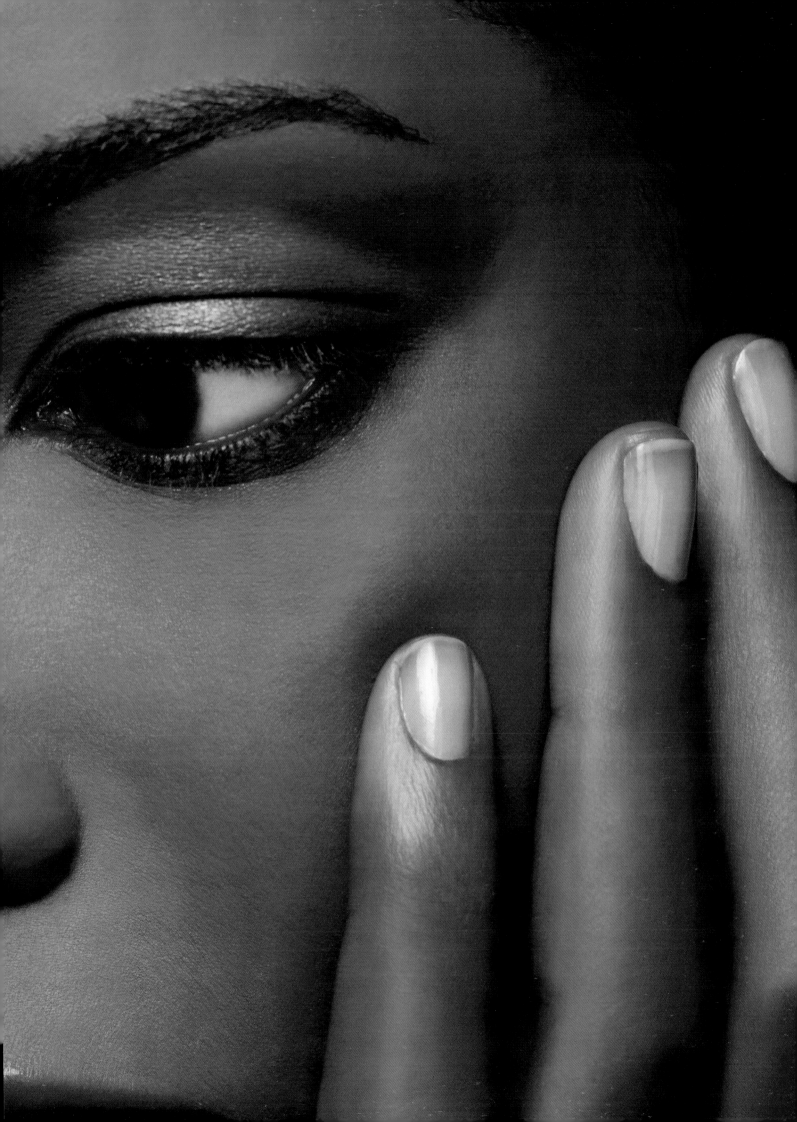

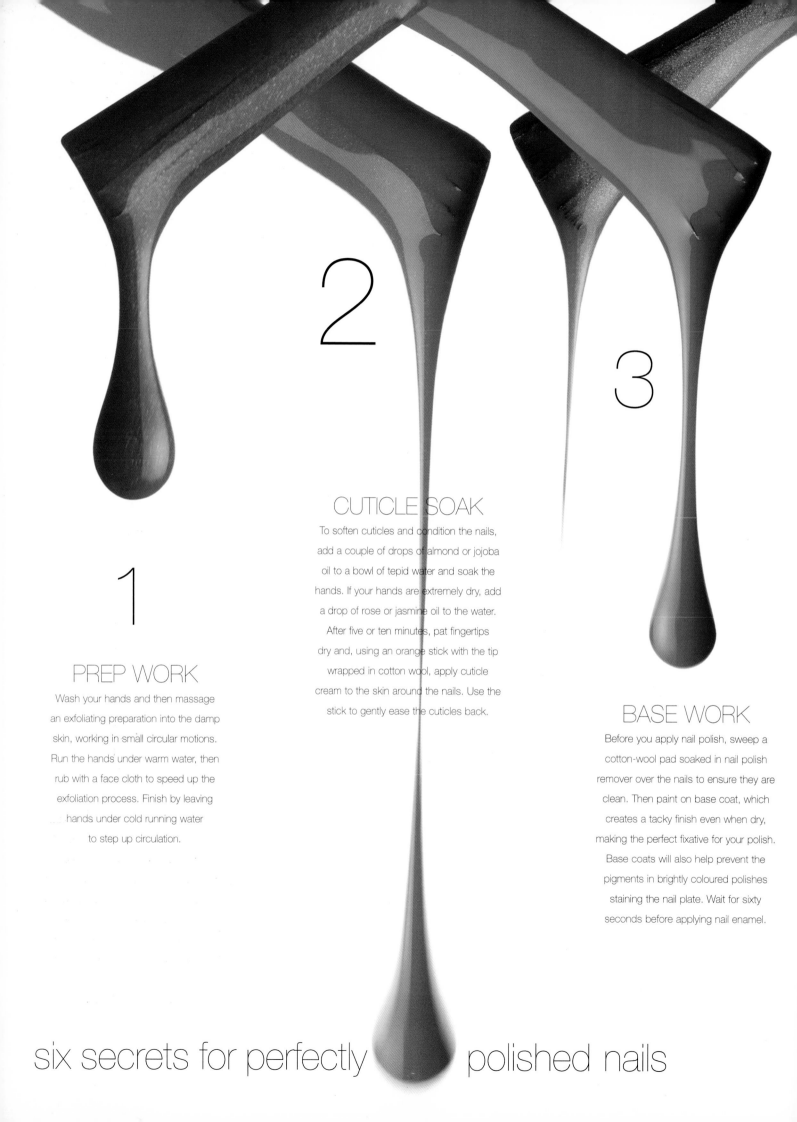

2

CUTICLE SOAK

To soften cuticles and condition the nails, add a couple of drops of almond or jojoba oil to a bowl of tepid water and soak the hands. If your hands are extremely dry, add a drop of rose or jasmine oil to the water. After five or ten minutes, pat fingertips dry and, using an orange stick with the tip wrapped in cotton wool, apply cuticle cream to the skin around the nails. Use the stick to gently ease the cuticles back.

3

1

PREP WORK

Wash your hands and then massage an exfoliating preparation into the damp skin, working in small circular motions. Run the hands under warm water, then rub with a face cloth to speed up the exfoliation process. Finish by leaving hands under cold running water to step up circulation.

BASE WORK

Before you apply nail polish, sweep a cotton-wool pad soaked in nail polish remover over the nails to ensure they are clean. Then paint on base coat, which creates a tacky finish even when dry, making the perfect fixative for your polish. Base coats will also help prevent the pigments in brightly coloured polishes staining the nail plate. Wait for sixty seconds before applying nail enamel.

six secrets for perfectly   polished nails

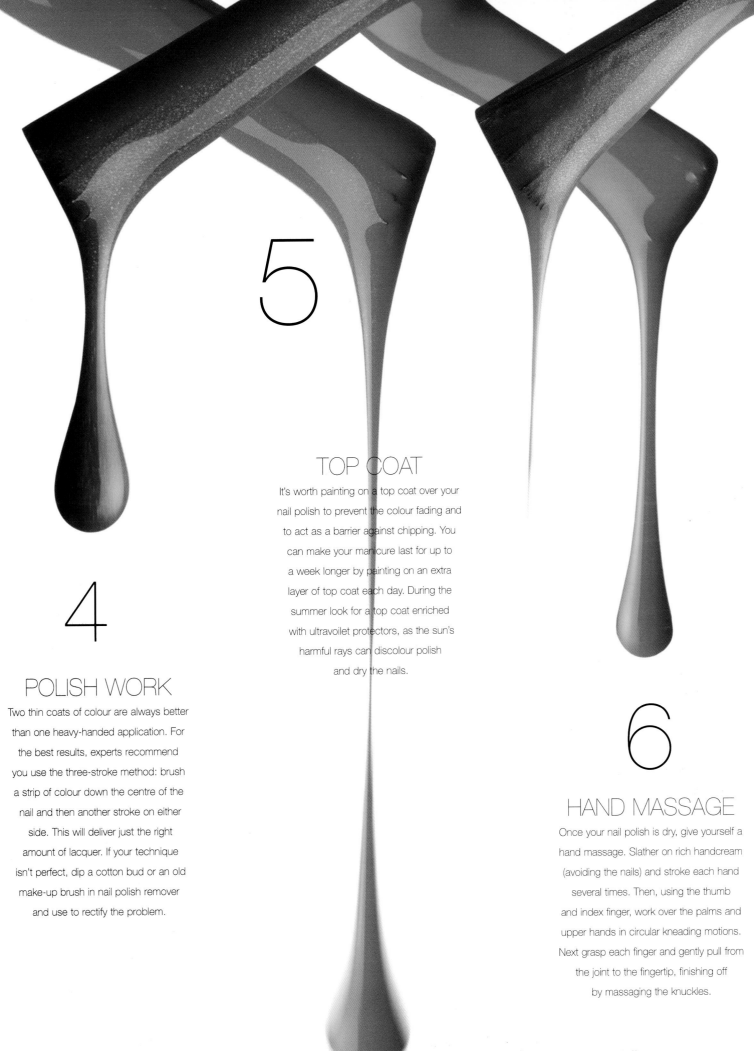

5

TOP COAT

It's worth painting on a top coat over your nail polish to prevent the colour fading and to act as a barrier against chipping. You can make your manicure last for up to a week longer by painting on an extra layer of top coat each day. During the summer look for a top coat enriched with ultravoilet protectors, as the sun's harmful rays can discolour polish and dry the nails.

4

POLISH WORK

Two thin coats of colour are always better than one heavy-handed application. For the best results, experts recommend you use the three-stroke method: brush a strip of colour down the centre of the nail and then another stroke on either side. This will deliver just the right amount of lacquer. If your technique isn't perfect, dip a cotton bud or an old make-up brush in nail polish remover and use to rectify the problem.

6

HAND MASSAGE

Once your nail polish is dry, give yourself a hand massage. Slather on rich handcream (avoiding the nails) and stroke each hand several times. Then, using the thumb and index finger, work over the palms and upper hands in circular kneading motions. Next grasp each finger and gently pull from the joint to the fingertip, finishing off by massaging the knuckles.

EYE WORK

EYEBROWS Incorrectly plucked brows will throw your face off balance. If you haven't plucked them before, leave it to the experts for the first time. You can then master tweezing as your brows regrow, using the initial shape as your guideline.

THE PERFECT ARCH Brows should always follow their natural shape. If you have small features, keep brows quite fine and tapered; if you have small, deep-set eyes, a well-shaped arch will make them appear bigger. To achieve the perfect arch, hold a pencil vertically alongside the nose to just above your brow bone: this is where the brows should start. Twist the pencil diagonally from the base of your nose to the outer corner of your eye: this is where your eyebrow should end. Then hold the pencil vertically to the outer corner of the iris: this is where the central edge of the arch should be. If you find it hard to shape the brows, draw in a guideline using an eye pencil before you start. This can be wiped off with cleanser afterwards.

TWEEZING Pluck hairs individually, clasping at the root and removing in the same direction as hair-growth. If you pluck too many hairs from the outer corners, this can make the eyes seem close-set; if you over-tweeze at the inner corners of the eyes, they will seem too far apart. Only remove stray hairs from beneath the brow bone and between the eyes. Plucking hairs above the brows can disturb the natural line and make the eyes appear smaller than they are. Be careful not to overpluck the brows as this can eventually prevent regrowth.

WAXING If you have extremely bushy brows or numerous hairs between the brows, you can have them waxed. It is a quick process, but should be done only by the experts and is more painful and expensive than tweezing. Hairs will grow back after about four to six weeks. To prevent ingrown hairs, gently massage an exfoliator into the brows at least once a week.

EYELASHES Apart from protecting them, eyelashes can really accentuate the eyes when they are curled and defined properly. With age, eyelashes tend to lose colour and become sparser, which makes it all the more important to define them.

CURLING Curling your eyelashes instantly opens up the eyes and adds definition to the face. Using metal lash curlers, clamp lashes near the roots, hold for several seconds and then release. Never curl mascara-laden lashes: as the mascara dries, lashes can stick to the curlers and be torn from the roots.

DYEING Having your eyelashes tinted professionally, or doing the job yourself at home, is worth considering if you do not like wearing mascara. If you decide on at-home dyeing, always put a thin film of Vaseline around the eye area first, as this will help stop dye staining the skin. You could use an old, clean mascara wand to make application easier. If you have sensitive eyes, it is not advisable to opt for eye-lash tinting. As you get older, avoid black dye, which can look harsh unless you have dark hair, and go for shades of brown, grey or dark blue.

PERMING Just like hair, eyelashes can be permanently curled. The process is similar, although the chemicals used are milder. Lashes are wrapped around a small rod while a perming solution is applied. The whole process is painless and usually takes an hour. Results remain true for up to a month.

FAKING IT Individual false lashes or strips cut to size can add definition. Run a small amount of clear lash glue along their edges, then, with a fingertip or tweezers, plant them by the roots of your natural lashes. To ease into place, use tweezers or an orange stick. If the glue shows, cover with mascara or liquid eyeliner. Coat false and natural lashes with mascara, to bind them together. Always remove false lashes before going to bed.

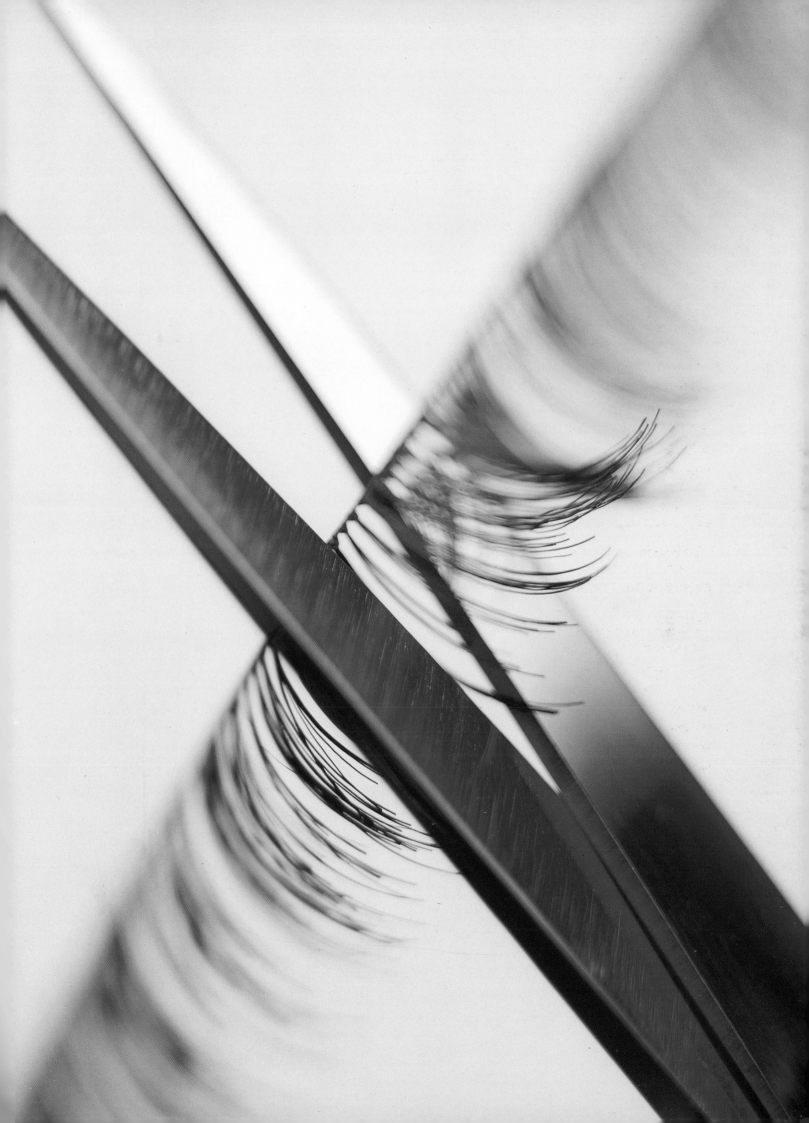

GOODGROOMING

FRESH-FACED

For those who want to look as though they are not wearing any foundation, but feel they need a helping hand to cover any imperfections, try mixing a small amount of foundation with your moisturizer. You can apply this liberally to the face and neck, sweeping it on in seconds. Make sure that the product does not collect in the eyebrows or under the eyes.

EYE RELIEF

Dark under-eye circles are either hereditary or caused by medication, stress, poor circulation or toxin build-up. To counteract, pat on stick concealer a shade lighter than skin tone. Puffy eyes can be caused by poor diet, sluggish lymph flow or the accumulation of toxins. Lay two chilled tablespoons (place briefly in freezer) on closed eyes as compresses.

SPOT FIX

A spot always seem to crop up when you're going somewhere special. If you can't resist picking, ensure that your hands are clean, use a tissue and gently squeeze the surrounding skin. Dab on tea tree or lavender oil – both antibacterial agents. To mask spots, paint concealer in the centre with a fine-tipped brush and gradually feather out, blending well, and set with powder.

LASH BOOST

If you're tired but want to look wide awake, add a couple of individual false lashes to the top outer corners of your eyelashes. Dip the end of each lash in clear lash glue, then plant the false lashes among the roots of your natural lashes. Once in place, hold until the glue sets. If the false lashes look like they are too long, trim to size before applying.

take short cuts to make yourself look good

LIP PRIMING
If you want a fresh-faced look with barely any make-up, ensure that your lips are in excellent condition. For an exfoliating treat, smooth on Vaseline and then very gently run a toothbrush over the lips. Alternatively, when you're exfoliating your face, work over the lips in circular motions with the fingertips – paying attention not to ingest any of the product!

FLATTERING FINISH
If your hands are not looking their best, this will affect your confidence and self-esteem. If you have sun and age spots or uneven skin tone on your hands, mix a long-lasting foundation with handcream and massage this into the skin. Afterwards, wipe the palms of your hands with a tissue to remove any of the product that has not been absorbed.

TRESS WORK
If your hair looks greasy but you have not got enough time to wash it, work with your hair's natural oils and simply add some wax or hair gel to slick the hair back, or sweep it up into a topknot. Alternatively, invest in a can of sprinkle-on dry shampoo to mask the greasiness. If time is not quite so pressing, wash hair with a combined shampoo and conditioner.

BROW DEFINITION
If you're not wearing make-up, but want to look good, groom your brows. Brush them up and then comb into place to remove stray hairs. If you have fair hair, give brows definition to strengthen your face. Dust on eyeshadow in a shade that matches your hair with a blunt-tipped brush or apply a pencil in small strokes and blend with the fingertips.

BEAUTY INTELLIGENCE

If you have sensitive skin, do not use any eye creams containing alpha hydroxy acids (AHAs) as they can cause irritation to the delicate areas around the eyes.

Avoid permanently tattooing in brow colour, which tends to look unnatural and can be a painful process. Instead, use a pencil to shape and define eyebrows.

If you find that your eyebrow hairs have become too long, you will need to trim their ends with a pair of nail scissors before you start work on your plucking.

If you have painted nails, avoid handcreams containing AHAs, which discolour polish. Instead, use a moisturizing face mask to hydrate the hands once a week.

You should always aim to tweeze your eyebrows after you've taken a bath or shower, since this is when the skin will be soft and at its most supple.

If you have had your hair lightened and want your brows to match, you can bleach them, but it's best to leave it to the experts to avoid a botched job.

Don't throw out old mascara wands. They can be cleaned with soap and warm water and then used to tame eyebrows or as an applicator for eyelash dye.

Every month you should stop wearing nail polish for at least four days, to allow air to get to the nail plate. Give nails a high-shine finish, using a nail buffer.

You should never use other people's mascara as this is one of the commonest ways of contracting conjunctivitis and spreading other eye infections.

Instead of mascara, make-up artists often use tinted brow-grooming gel to define the lashes, as this adds thickness and colour but still looks natural.

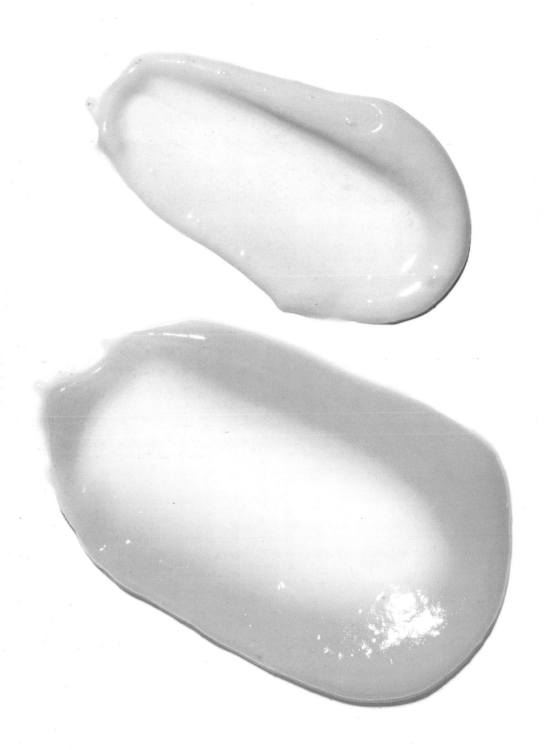

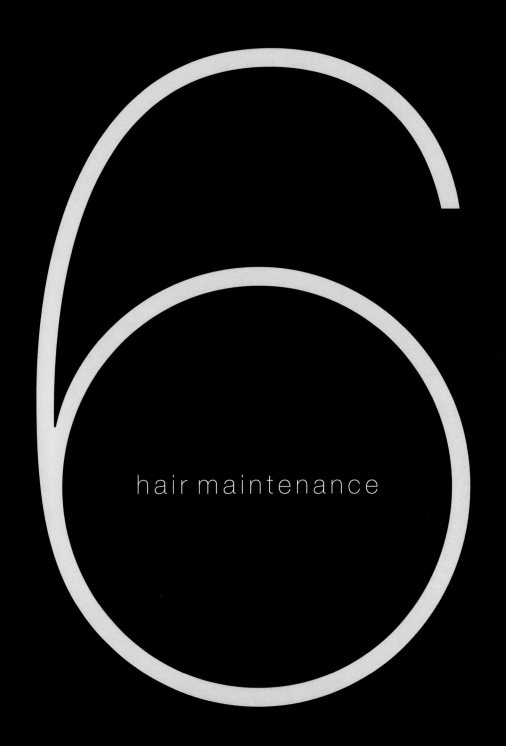

hair maintenance

Everyone can have great hair, even those of us not naturally blessed with thick, lustrous tresses. The secrets behind maintaining healthy-looking hair lie in combining the right maintenance regime with the appropriate products, and then in following professional advice. After that, keeping your hair in perfect condition should be quick and easy.

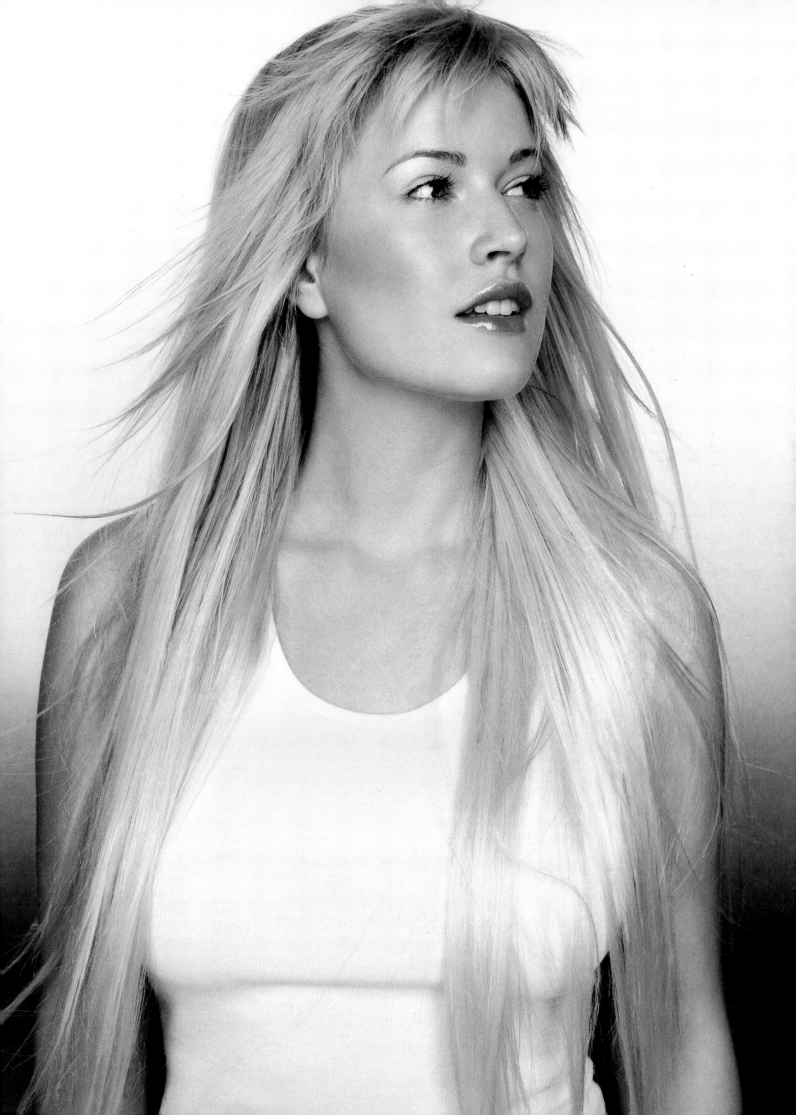

HAIR-CARE ESSENTIALS

LEAVE-IN CONDITIONER

is a no-rinse option for conditioning the hair and is ideal if you are pushed for time. It won't weigh fine hair down and helps tame flyaway, frizzy hair. If the ends of your hair are extremely dry, you can smooth a small amount of leave-in conditioner on as a post styling fix. This will help hydrate and protect the ends, whilst improving their appearance.

SHAMPOOS

are detergent-based, alkaline and work by swelling the hair shaft and lifting the cuticle. They also carry an electric charge which causes individual hair strands to react with one another, producing static. After shampooing, hair is left with a negative charge and the cuticles will be dishevelled; conditioners contain positively charged agents that bond with the negative charge of the hair.

CONDITIONER

should always be used after shampooing. Designed to work within thirty to sixty seconds, it makes the cuticles surrounding the hair shaft lie flat, creating an even surface to reflect light, making the hair appear shiny and glossy. If you shave your legs, get more mileage from hair conditioner by smoothing it on to damp skin whilst in the bath or shower to shave the legs. It ensures a smooth shave and helps keep the skin's moisture content topped up.

SCALP TONICS

may be required from time to time when your scalp is out of condition. To check your scalp, make a parting down the centre of your head; if there is any scaling, it needs attention. Don't automatically assume you have dandruff, the problem could be a dry scalp, which can be treated by massaging with almond oil, or it could be sunburn, or a build-up of styling preparation. Wash with your regular shampoo and then take another look. If the problem remains, treat with a scalp tonic.

DETOXING SHAMPOOS

have been created to remove the build-up of city dirt, styling preparations and chlorine. They contain higher concentrations of cleansers than normal shampoos and increased levels of chelators, which bind to the surface of the hair to remove collected minerals. For the best results substitute your regular shampoo with a detoxing or clarifying formula every five to seven washes, lather up, leave for a couple of minutes

HAIR MASKS

should be used once a week if your hair feels dry or is damaged from heat styling, chemical processing or sun exposure. To step up the conditioning properties of a hair mask, wrap the head in cling film or wear a shower cap and blast with the hair dryer. The heat will enhance the activity of the conditioning ingredients and allow for better absorption of the product.

HAIR TYPES

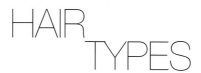

NORMAL If you are lucky enough to have been blessed with normal hair, look after it. Wash and condition it every two to three days, or whenever necessary. Just because your hair is normal, this doesn't mean it's more resilient. Take measures to maintain overall condition by using products which will protect it from heat styling and shield it from ultraviolet light. Have trims regularly to help prevent split ends. There is nothing to stop most people achieving normal hair if they look after it sensibly.

DRY If your hair is dry, it is not receiving sufficient oil from the scalp. This can be the result of exposure to the sun, stress, dietary imbalances and chemical processing (such as colouring or perming), or a hereditary condition. Try using moisturizing shampoos and conditioners to hydrate the hair. Give the scalp a pre-cleansing treat by massaging with almond or jojoba oil (which is similar to the hair's natural oil). Leave oil on for about ten minutes before shampooing. Brush your hair regularly to stimulate the scalp and to distribute the existing oils throughout.

GREASY Greasy hair is caused by overactive sebaceous glands which produce too much oil, known as sebum. Stress, poor diet, hormonal imbalances and harsh hair-care products can trigger the glands to go into overdrive. To remedy this, wash your hair daily with a mild shampoo, making sure that you cleanse the scalp effectively, and use a lightweight conditioner. Once a week, try rubbing jojoba oil (which is similar to the hair's natural oil) into the scalp and leave it on overnight. Adding oil like this will trick the hair into believing that it is producing the oil itself and so will help regulate the natural sebum production.

CHEMICALLY TREATED Perming or colouring changes the hair's porosity, making it more susceptible to damage. You should always use shampoos and conditioners which are specially formulated for chemically treated hair – they will have been designed to maintain either the colour or the curl of the hair. Use protein-enriched hair masks to help strengthen and repair the hair; these work by bonding to the hair shaft where the damage has occurred during chemical processing. Colour-treated hair fades in the sun, so you should really wear a hat, or at least use products that contain sun protectors.

COMBINATION It is very common to have active sebaceous glands which make the scalp and the roots of the hair greasy while the mid-lengths and ends are dry, frizzy and prone to breakage. To deal with this problem, you don't need to splash out on a wide range of shampoos and conditioners. Instead, massage a mild shampoo into the roots, where grease accumulates and attracts dirt, and run through the rest of the hair. Finish by working conditioner into the mid-lengths and the ends of the hair (avoiding the roots and scalp). Never have the water too hot, as this will stimulate the oil-producing glands.

BLACK HAIR Black hair is usually coarse and dry, making it susceptible to damage and breakage, and as a result it can be hard to handle. You should use intensive pre-shampoo treatments to help hydrate the scalp and the hair, massage the scalp regularly to encourage oil production, shampoo as often as necessary and only lather once. Give the hair a hot-oil treatment once a month. If you feel you want to tame very curly Afro hair, try demi-perming, which will transform tight curls into larger, looser ones. The hair is woven on to rollers to redefine the shape. To maintain, you should use special curl activators and moisturizing sprays. Straightening or relaxing is another option for Afro hair. This is a chemical process which has the reverse effect to perming. Chemical relaxers are made in different strengths to suit different hair textures and styles.

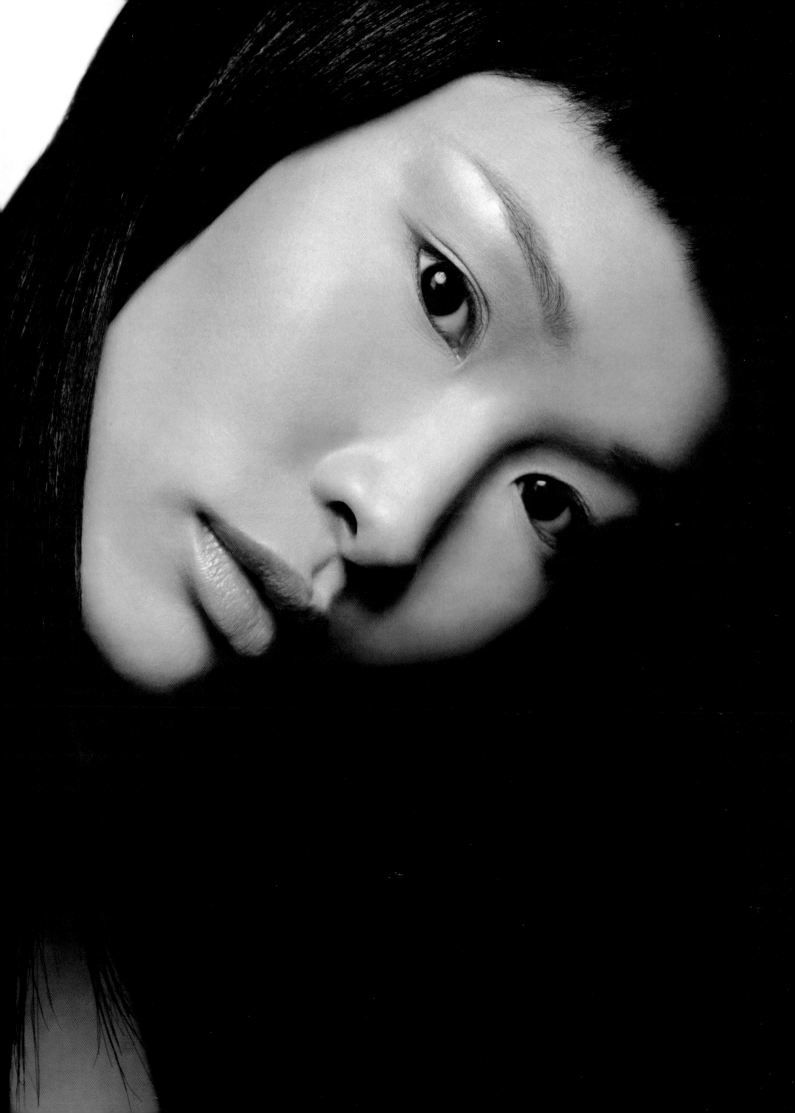

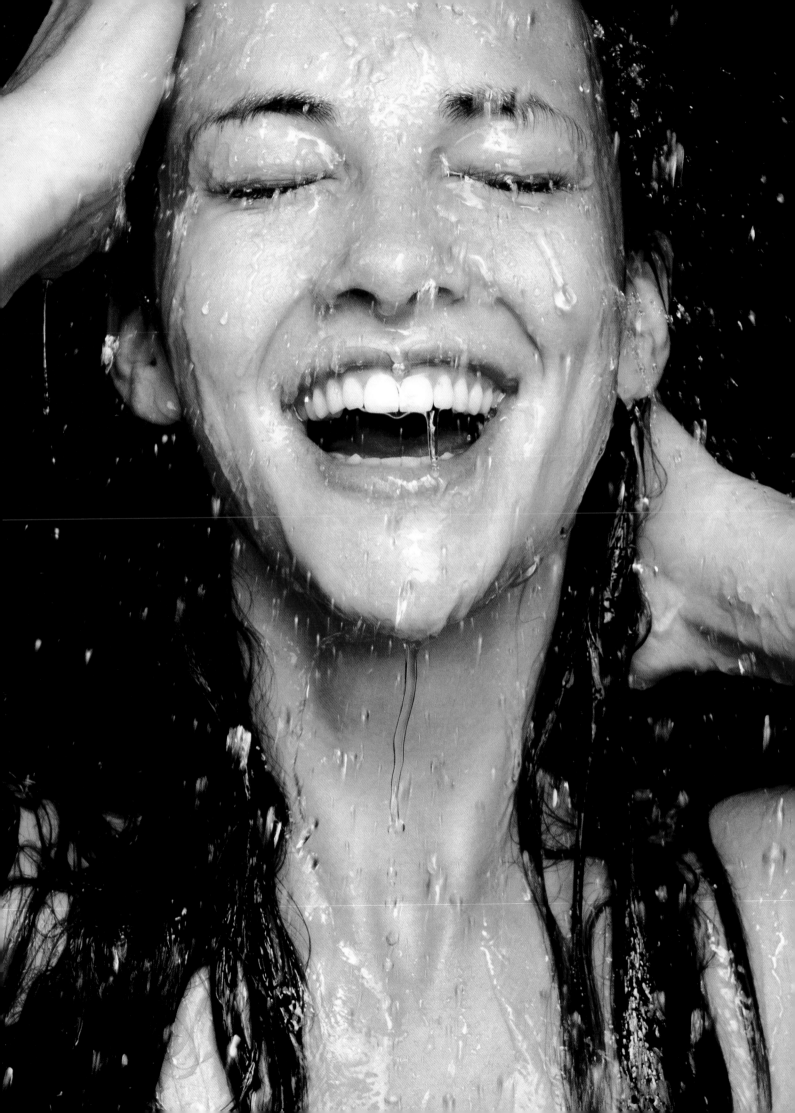

HAIR UPKEEP

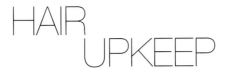

CLEANSING Either look for a shampoo that is suited to your hair type or invest in a very mild formulation. If your shampoo doesn't lather to a mass of suds and bubbles, this is not an indication that it will not cleanse the hair thoroughly. In fact, as the amount of suds is determined by the active level of detergent, many shampoos that do not lather are more effective. Never use too much shampoo, as over-washing will remove the hair's natural oils. Do not wash hair with washing-up liquid, soap or other detergents, as they are very alkaline and can disrupt the natural balance of the hair. You should change your shampoo every few months, as the hair will develop a resistance to certain ingredients after a period of time. Never wash your hair in dirty bath water; despite the temptation to save time this way, it won't clean the hair properly. You should wash your hair every two to three days to avoid the build-up of dirt and sebum that can create a breeding ground for bacteria, leading to dullness, dandruff and a flaky scalp. If you wash your hair daily, one shampoo will suffice; if you insist on washing it twice, use only a small amount of shampoo. Keep the water tepid when you are washing your hair, as hot water can agitate the scalp and step up the activity of the oil-producing glands, making hair greasy. Before applying conditioner, blot excess moisture from the hair with a towel or squeeze with the hands.

CONDITIONING Conditioners play a vital role in maintaining the shine and general appearance of the hair. If you skip them, it can result in your cuticles not lying flat and your hair looking dull and lifeless. It will also be more susceptible to damage. Conditioning sprays are a cross between leave-in conditioners and styling preparations, making them ideal for people with short hair or those who don't want to spend too long on their hair-care regimes. You need to apply conditioner only to the mid-lengths and ends of the hair, as the scalp's oil-producing glands usually supply the roots with sufficient moisture. After applying, run a wide-toothed comb gently through the hair, rinse thoroughly and finish with a blast of cold water. This ensures that the cuticles will lie flat and provides a stimulating boost for the scalp. Do not towel-dry the hair vigorously but simply blot off any excess water; otherwise you will damage the hair and dishevel the cuticles. Never brush the hair when it is wet, always using a wide-toothed comb instead.

SCALP WORK When the hair is wet, treat your scalp to a massage. Use warm olive oil if your scalp feels dry or tight; go for equal amounts of witch hazel and mineral water if you have an oily scalp; and mix equal amounts of rose water and mineral water if your scalp is normal. Using the pads of the fingertips, start at the forehead and gently rotate around the hairline. Move to the sides and work over the crown to the nape of the neck. This kneading motion will pep up the blood supply and increase the flow of nutrients and oxygen to the hair follicles. It will also help reduce scalp tension – one cause of hair loss – and help stabilize over-active sebaceous glands.

HAIR MASKS If your hair is dry and damaged from chemical processing, excessive heat styling or sun exposure, incorporate a deep-conditioning hair mask into your beauty regime until your locks are restored to their former glory. You will have to use your own judgement when deciding how often to go for this type of mask, bearing in mind that one of the commonest causes of lifeless-looking hair is over-conditioning. Protein masks rebuild the hair, as they are absorbed into the cuticle, strengthening the hair shaft, while moisturizing packs help hydrate and improve manageability. For the best results, use on freshly washed hair which has been blotted with a towel to remove excess water. To step up the conditioning properties of a hair mask, slather on before going into a sauna or steam room. If you're heading for the beach, it's a good idea to smooth on a hair mask, leaving the sun to activate the ingredients. This will protect your hair and also improve its overall condition.

FLAKY SCALP

Often confused with dandruff, flaky scalp occurs when surface skin cells come away. This can result from poor circulation, not brushing the hair sufficiently, using harsh products and not rinsing shampoo off properly. To treat, use a mild or moisturizing shampoo, working into the scalp thoroughly. If the scalp is not meticulously clean, it is a perfect breeding ground for bacteria. Shampooing will lift dead skin cells, but if application is too rapid they will only flake off when the scalp and hair dry. Avoid medicated shampoos, which tend to work only temporarily as they can contain ingredients that irritate the scalp.

DANDRUFF

Dandruff appears as thick greasy patches on the scalp which can easily become infected, resulting in scabbing and inflammation. This type of dandruff (seborrheic dermatitis), usually linked with a food allergy or poor diet, is aggravated by stress or excessive intake of dairy products and junk foods. Wash the hair daily with a shampoo formulated for dandruff or blend ten drops of thyme essential oil with 100ml of apple juice, massage into the scalp, leave for five minutes, rinse the hair and then use a mild shampoo. Take four 500mg capsules of evening primrose oil every day until the condition clears.

ECZEMA RELIEF

If you have red patches on your scalp which are itchy, it's likely that you have eczema or psoriasis. If you're unsure, consult a trichologist or your hairdresser or doctor. Use a mild or moisturizing shampoo (avoid medicated formulas, which contain ingredients which can irritate the scalp). Wash hair daily, then massage pure aloe vera juice or cold camomile tea into the scalp, leave on and style as normal. If you have very fine hair, use this remedy as an overnight treatment and rinse out in the morning, as it can weigh the hair down, making it hard to handle. Try cutting out dairy foods to see if things improve.

TEMPORARY HAIR LOSS

On average it is normal to lose 100 hairs each day. Temporary hair loss can also occur after pregnancy, and as a result of stress, taking medication or illness, but the hair usually grows back. Unless you are pregnant, treat the scalp as follows: blend two drops each of basil and rosemary essential oils with 10ml of avocado oil, place in a glass bottle and gently heat in a bowl of near-boiling water, then massage into the scalp and wait thirty minutes before shampooing. Traction hair loss is caused by braiding or weaving hair too tightly too often, which can disrupt hair follicles, causing scar tissue to form.

HEREDITARY HAIR LOSS

This condition affects some 10 per cent of all women. There are many treatments on offer, but they are expensive, can have unpleasant side effects and do not live up to their claims. New research has suggested ways to help prevent the onset of hereditary hair loss. As we age, the collagen on the scalp will harden and accumulate, eventually strangling the hair follicles. As a result of this, all hair growth is stopped. New preparations are available to reduce the collagen build-up. If hair loss runs in the family, take preventive steps by eating foods rich in biotin, which can be found in cauliflower and nuts.

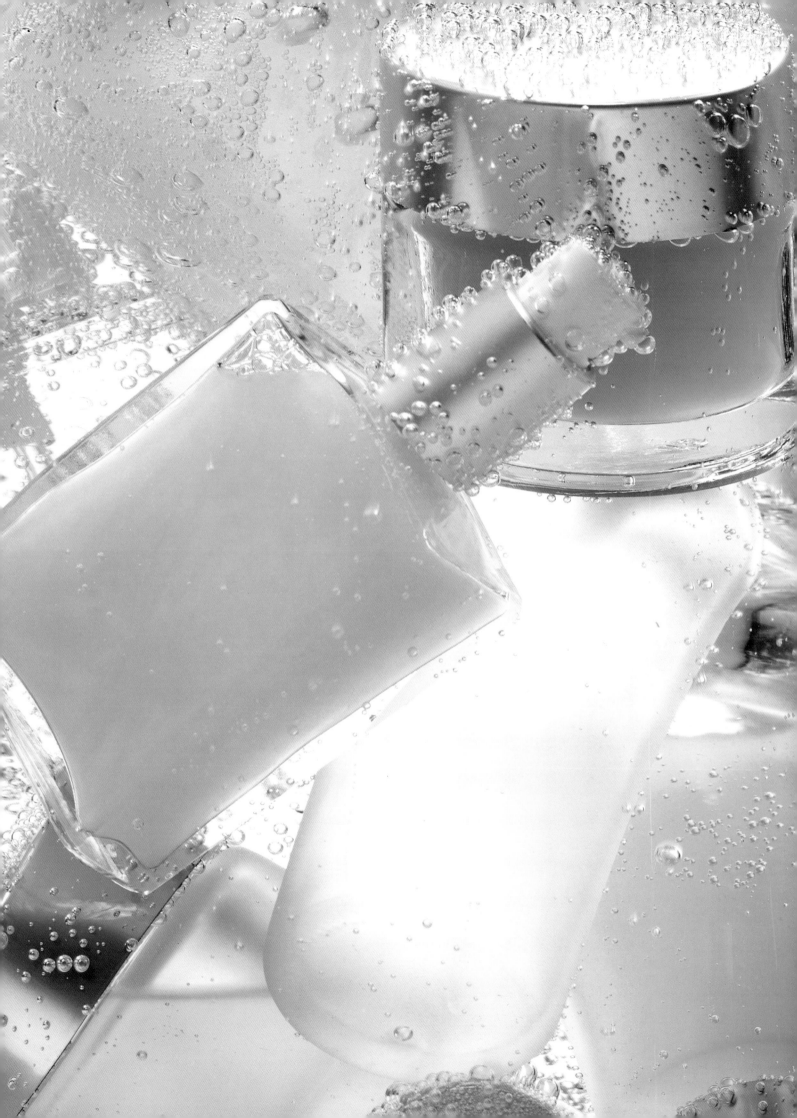

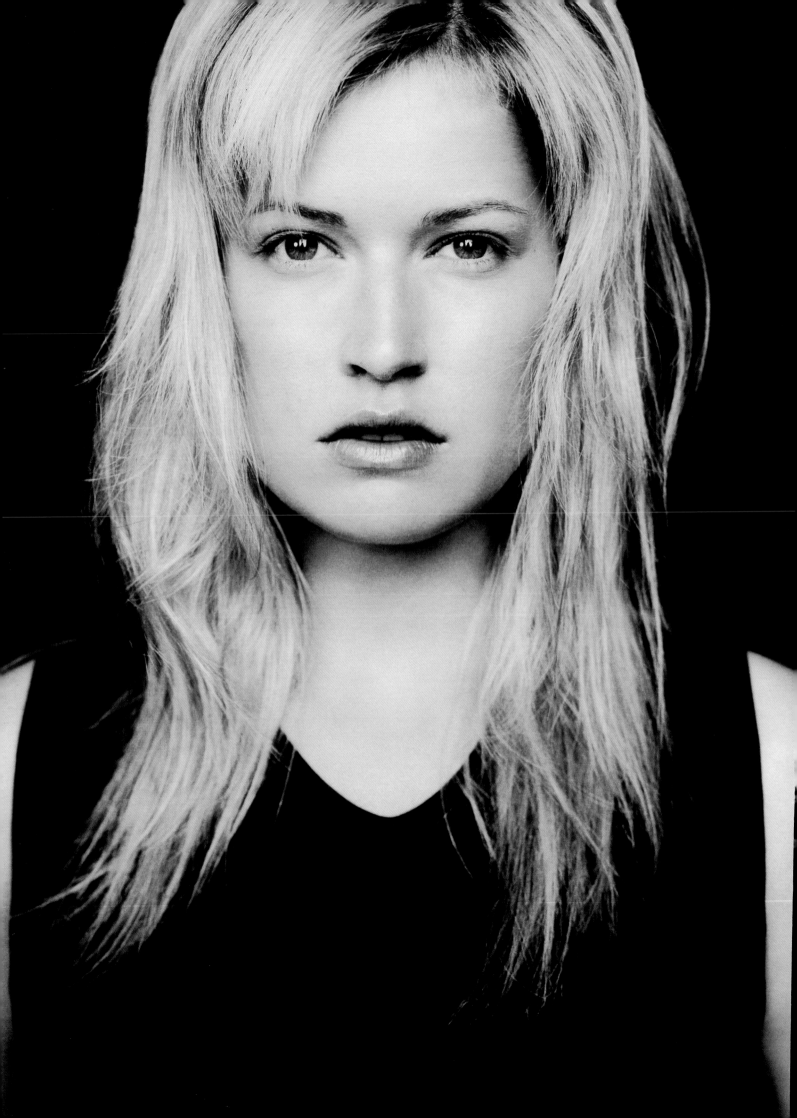

PREGNANCY

Hormonal changes during pregnancy will affect skin and hair. For the first three months, sebaceous glands can be over-active, leading to oily hair, so use mild shampoo daily. Thereafter, hair has a prolonged growth period, so is thick and shiny. Avoid excessive chemical processing now. Many aromatherapy oils can be harmful if you're pregnant, so check product ingredients. After the birth, as hormones readapt, hair can seem dull and hair loss excessive, but this is just hair that would have been lost earlier. Take wheatgerm or brewer's yeast, natural sources of vitamin B that is important for healthy hair.

FRIZZY HAIR

Atmospheric moisture can be a nightmare, turning the sleekest locks into a frizzy mess. To overcome this, look for styling preparations that repel moisture – serums and pomades are a good choice. Alternatively, try using a leave-in conditioner after shampooing. It won't overload the hair but will help retain moisture and prevent frizz. To style the hair and help repel moisture, hairdressers advise mixing equal amounts of hair gel and serum and then applying. Alternatively, stop fighting the frizz and adapt your hairstyle instead: try scrunching gel into your hair to encourage natural movement and give it body.

STATIC HAIR

All strands of hair have an electrical charge which is positive or negative. When either two positive or two negative hair strands repel each other, it makes the hair go static. This can occur as a result of the friction created when brushing or blow-drying the hair, or when you pull an item of clothing on over your head. Conditioners, mousse and styling sprays can help to restore the electrical balance, keeping your hair soft and static-free. If you are looking for a quick way to tame static hair, you could try applying a fine mist of hairspray to your hairbrush or comb and then gently running it through flyaway hair.

OIL SLICK

Taking medication, stress, poor diet, hormonal imbalances and harsh products can throw your scalp's oil-producing glands into a state of flux. One of the simplest solutions to the problem is to not wash your hair. After three days, oil production will slow down and your hair will begin to look healthy and shiny. Instead of washing it, rinse the hair daily first with warm water, then with cool water. This trick works wonders for thick and curly or permed hair and colour-treated hair (the colour won't fade so quickly), but can be disastrous if your hair is fine, leaving you with lank and greasy-looking locks.

DULL HAIR

This can result from bad circulation, build-up of styling preparations, harsh shampoos or poor diet. To make hair lustrous, increase your intake of pantothenic acid, found in wheatgerm, peanuts and egg yolks. After shampooing, rinse with the juice of a lemon (or a capful of vinegar) diluted in a litre of cold water. The acidity flattens the cuticles, leaving your hair shiny. Hairdressers advise adding serum to the hair, then running a large make-up brush down the hair shaft to smooth cuticles and give hair a polished finish. Curly hair can look dull, as the cuticles don't lie flat – try a leave-in conditioner or conditioning spray.

UNDER ATTACK

SUN EXPOSURE

Ultraviolet rays damage the hair, alter its colour and can burn the scalp. To strengthen the hair and make it more resilient to UV attack, prepare yourself a couple of months before heading for the sun. Start with regular conditioning treatments and have your haircut adapted so it requires less maintenance and less heat styling. Use hair-care products and styling preparations which contain UV protectors – look for products with Parsol MCX (a UV filter) on the label. Wearing a hat is one of the safest ways to protect the hair and scalp, and can also reduce the risks of heatstroke. During the summer or after sun exposure, hair will become drier and more susceptible to damage. To keep the moisture content up, swap your regular shampoo for a moisturizing formula. Unless your hair is extremely dry, it is not advisable to change to a moisturizing conditioner, which can overload the hair, making it look dull and lank. Instead treat dry and brittle hair with a more intensive treatment once a week. Cut back on the use of heat-styling appliances during the summer to help maintain condition. Leave your hair to dry naturally. The warmth of the air will speed up the process; hair will be 75 per cent dry in fifteen minutes in the summer. To finish, use a hair-dryer on a cool setting. When you are in the sun, don't scrape the hair up into a topknot, as this exposes the ends of the hair to the sun's harmful rays. Instead sweep hair back to the nape of the neck, thus shielding the skin from the sun, hiding ends which are susceptible to damage and allowing for an even colour fade.

WATER IRRITATION

The chemicals and impurities in chlorinated and salt water can play havoc with the colour and condition of the hair. If you have dry, damaged or colour-treated hair, it is advisable to use a water-resistant or waterproof hair-protection product before you go swimming. The water-resistant ingredients are locked into the product until the hair comes into contact with water, at which point the oils are released and immediately adhere to the hair, protecting it and stopping it from drying out. If you swim in chlorinated or salt water, you should always wash your hair as soon as you come out. After swimming in the sea, if there is no alternative, you can rinse your hair with carbonated mineral water or soda water.

POLLUTION PERILS

Smoke, city grime and other pollutants can collect on the hair, making it look dull and lifeless. Other by-products from cigarette smoke and natural gas from cookers can also discolour the hair – they are said to give white hair a yellowish tinge. To remove such a build-up, use clarifying, purifying or chelating shampoos, all of which contain a high concentration of cleansers to shift stubborn dirt and will also ensure that there are no mineral residues left on the hair. If you find your hair smells of smoke or unpleasant cooking odours and you do not have time to wash it, spray a fine mist of perfume on to your comb or brush and run it through your hair.

WEATHER EXTREMES

Just as the wind, central heating and air conditioning have a drying effect on the skin, they can also play havoc with the hair, making it very brittle. You should use a more intensive conditioner or a leave-in conditioner to combat dryness caused by cold weather. In freezing temperatures the hair picks up static electricity, becoming flyaway and hard to handle. You can reduce the static charge by spraying a hairbrush or comb with hairspray and gently running it through the hair. Central heating draws moisture from the hair and the scalp, which can also result in static. To reduce the drying effects of central heating, place large bowls of water near the radiators or use humidifiers. If you are in the snow, remember that the sun's rays are intensified by the reflection of the snow, so your hair will need extra protection.

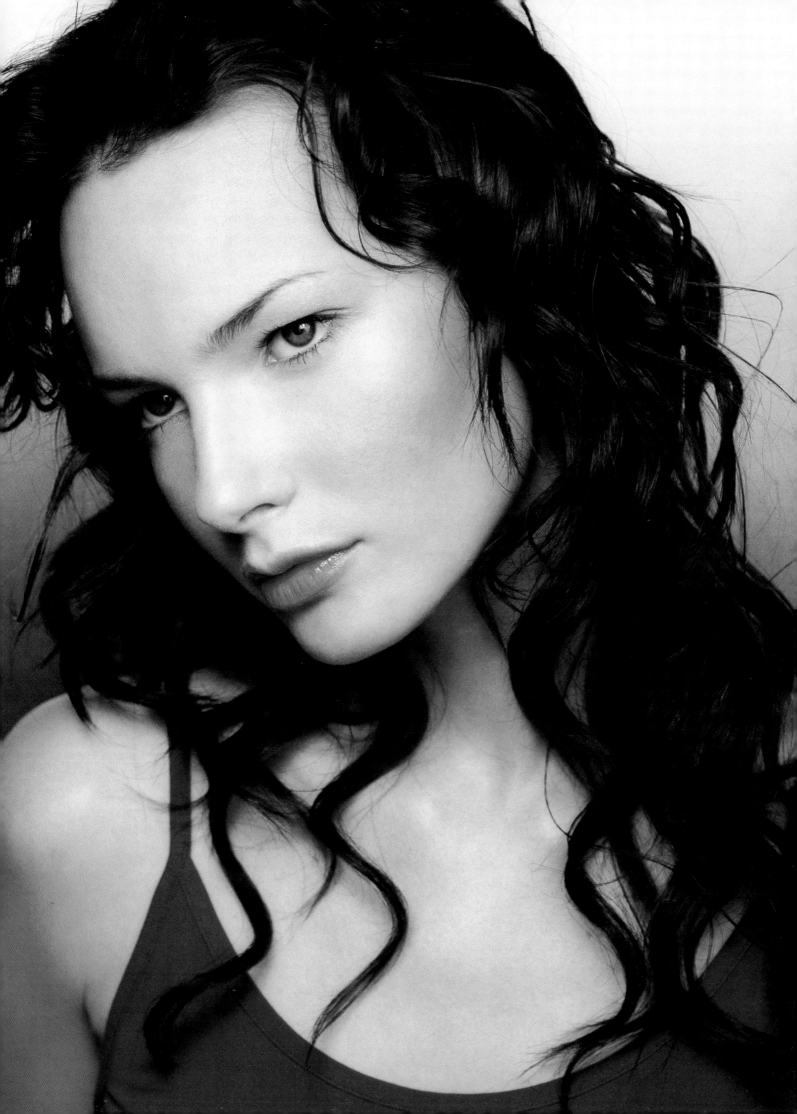

HAIRCYCLE

GROWTH PHASES

Hair grows about 12mm a month and each strand has three growth phases before being replaced by a new hair. If it is not cut, hair strands will grow to 107cm before being shed. Over time, growth decreases. To maintain healthy growth, massage the scalp regularly in order to stimulate the flow of nutrients, oxygen and blood to the hair follicles.

TEXTURE TURNS

It is inevitable that our hair's texture will change. The great body and volume that we experienced during adolescence will start to diminish and hair will become thinner and finer as it loses a third of its original diameter. However, clever cutting techniques, modern perms and body-building styling preparations mean none of this should pose a problem.

COLOUR CHANGES

As we age, hair loses its natural colour: blonde hair fades, red hair tones down to shades with brown undertones and brunettes lose their natural highlights. This is because the activity of the hair's colour-producing cells decreases and eventually stops over time (sometimes early in life). Hairs will then be white, and not grey, as commonly perceived.

CONDITION ISSUE

The overall condition of the hair will change with time. From an early age, the sebaceous glands will be at their most active, but gradually the production of the hair's natural oils slows down and hair will become drier and feel coarser. To overcome this, step up the use of conditioning preparations and use a hair mask once a week.

adapt your hair-care regime to suit your age

STRESS OUT

Work-related stress takes its toll on the hair and scalp. This can start during your twenties and will manifest itself through a dry, flaky scalp or the appearance of bald patches which usually regrow. If you lead a stressful life, step up your intake of B viitamins, found in wholegrain cereals, oily fish, yeast extracts, peas, natural yoghurt, eggs and milk.

HAIR FOOD

Current research has shown that a fat-free diet can affect the condition of your hair, causing it to look dull and lifeless, and can also result in a dry scalp. If your hair suddenly becomes dry, it is advisable to increase your intake of essential fatty acids. These can be found in vegetable oils, in nuts and in oily fish, such as sardines, red mullet, and salmon.

FRAME WORK

As you get older, if you wear glasses choose frames and a hairstyle that complement each other. Always take your glasses to the salon, so your hairdresser can see what you look like with them on. Remember, large glasses will seem out of place with neat feather cuts, while thin-framed, small glasses will seem unbalanced with masses of curls.

HORMONAL CHANGES

Our hormones play a vital role in the condition of our hair. Women may experience temporary hair loss while taking or coming off the pill and those on HRT may notice an improvement in the hair's texture and condition. During pregnancy hair will become drier as increased oestrogen production decreases sebum levels, but will look thicker.

BEAUTY INTELLIGENCE

1 Don't be fooled into thinking shampoos and conditioners loaded with vitamins are better for your hair – with the exception of B5, they can't be absorbed.

2 A strand of healthy hair should be able to stretch up to 30 per cent of its normal length before breaking. Healthy hair will grow on average 15cm each year.

3 Remember, you can always get some extra mileage from your shampoo when you are on the move by using it to wash your body and even your clothes too.

4 Brush tangled hair from the ends, working your way slowly to the roots, or you will have knots throughout. Work gently to avoid ripping the hair shaft.

5 If the skin on your knees and elbows is dry but you have no moisturizer to hand, massage a small amount of creamy hair conditioner into the skin instead.

Condition dry, damaged hair by applying a protein hair mask, then blasting with a hair-dryer. Heat helps active ingredients get to work far more effectively.

Never rinse your hair in dirty bath water, as it will probably contain alkaline soap residues which will cling to the hair, making it dull and lifeless-looking after styling.

If your hair feels rough when you finish shampooing, this could be an indication that the shampoo you are using is too harsh and not suitable for your type of hair.

If you have coloured your hair, you should avoid using anti-dandruff shampoos, as these have been found to accelerate colour fade in some instances.

If you have fine hair, use a volumizing spray containing polymers before blow-drying. The heat will swell the polymers, making the hair appear thicker.

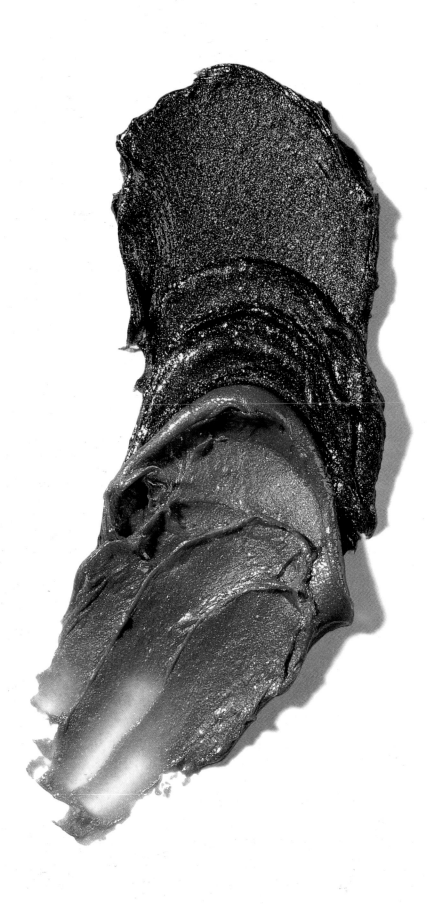

prep work

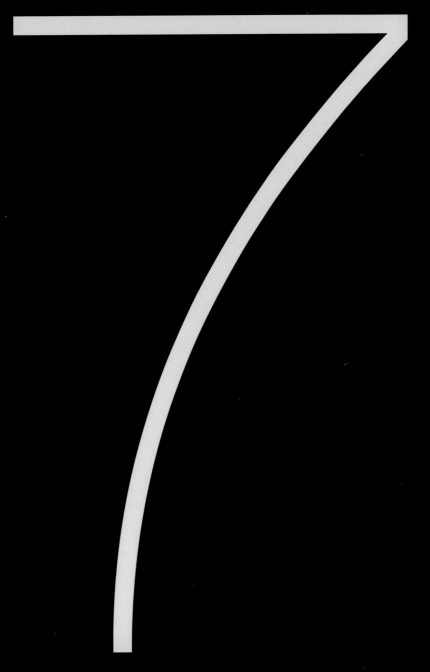

Provided that you choose a haircut which complements the shape of your face, you find styling products which work in harmony with your hair type, and you use the appliances which make light work of styling, there is no reason why you cannot keep your hair looking great all the time. These are the secrets of successful hair-styling.

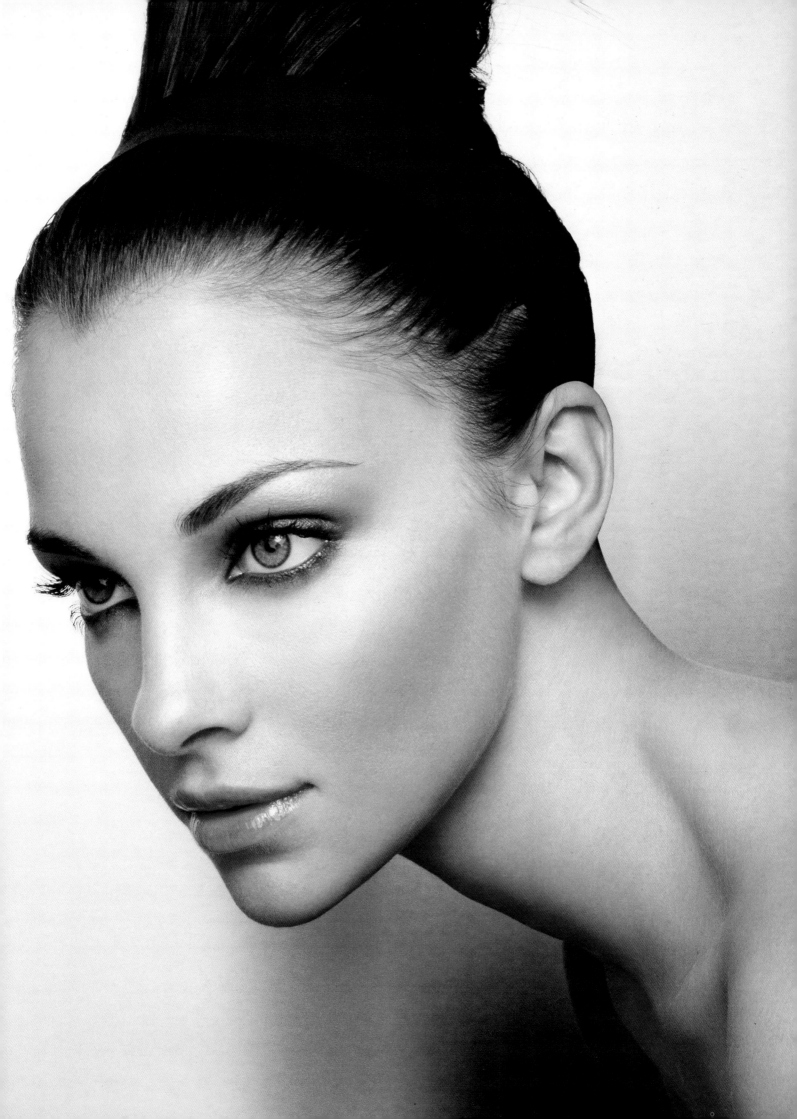

STYLING
ESSENTIALS

WAX

is ideal for adding texture to
short styles and definition to curly hair.
To tame unruly hairs around the face or
to redefine curls, look for a lightweight
formula, and then use a heavier wax on
shorter styles or to break up thick hair.
Apply sparingly, rubbing a small amount
into the palms of the hands and then
running hands through hair. Never
apply wax to roots or fine hair.

MOUSSE

gives body to most styles, but works
best on fine hair, creating good hold
without stickiness. For root lift, apply to
the palms, rub together and massage
into the roots before blow-drying. To add
body, apply to the mid-lengths and ends,
comb through and blow-dry. For more
hold, don't use more product but buy a
formulation with extra-holding properties.

SETTING LOTION

or styling sprays contain flexible resins
that form a film on the hair and help with
styling, while preventing heat damage.
Look for a formulation suited to your
particular hair type. Add to the roots if
root lift is required or smooth on to the
mid-lengths and ends. Take care not to
use too much, as it can make the hair
look dull and feel unpleasant.

HAIRSPRAY

is used as a finishing preparation to keep hair in place. Shake the can well and then spray on, holding it at least 12cm from your head. Apply sparingly, as too much can weigh the hair down. For a post-styling fix to smooth stray cuticles, spray a brush or comb with a fine mist of hairspray and then run it over the hair shaft. Avoid using sprays containing alcohol if you have dry hair.

SERUM

is usually silicone-based and forms a microscopic film on the surface of the hair shaft to enhance shine and softness. Apply sparingly – two or three drops are enough – or hair can look greasy. Use on wet hair to deal with tangles or scrunch into curls to reduce frizz and combat static, or smooth down the hair shaft to tame unruly cuticles or use to temporarily seal split ends.

POMADES

are softer than waxes and do not weigh the hair down so much. Use to slick hair back, smooth cuticles and add definition to short styles. Apply sparingly and avoid altogether if you have fine hair. Anti-humectant pomades help prevent hair going frizzy in humid conditions, forming a moisture-repellent shield on the hair shaft.

GEL

is available in different consistencies, ranging from lightweight sprays to thicker jelly types. Use on wet hair to protect before blow-drying and add volume, or on dry styles to slick the hair back or to add texture to shorter styles. If gel dries on the hair and feels brittle, mix with a small amount of serum before applying.

BRUSH WORK

Brushing your hair will help smooth the cuticles, enhancing shine, will stimulate the blood supply to hair follicles, promoting healthy growth, and will remove accumlated dirt and dead skin cells. Always brush the hair before shampooing to make the hair tangle-free. Forget anything you may have been told about the need to brush your hair a hundred strokes a day before you go to bed – in fact, over-zealous brushing can tear the hair and is likely to remove far too many of its natural oils.

BRISTLE CHOICE
Choose a hairbrush to suit your particular hair type and styling requirements. Brushes with natural bristles are less damaging to the hair, but natural bristles alone will be too soft to penetrate wet or thick hair, which needs the added strength supplied by a mix of nylon and natural bristles. For thick, curly hair, a brush with closely spaced, all-nylon bristles will offer maximum control for smoothing or straightening; widely spaced bristles will minimize pull to enhance wave and volume. For fine or thinning hair, use a soft-bristle brush. For Afro hair that has been relaxed, use a natural-bristle brush and for curly styles use a wide-toothed Afro comb.

THE RIGHT BRUSH
Flat brushes, usually oval or rectangular in shape, are ideal for basic work to smooth and untangle the hair. Paddle brushes have large, flat bases, making them suitable for longer-length hair. Vent brushes have vented, hollow centres to allow a heated stream of air to flow through the brush and the hair, thus ensuring high-speed drying and making light work of root lift or adding volume in almost any style. They are especially good for blow-drying relaxed Afro hair. For straightening curly hair, smoothing the sleeker styles or styling short hair, round brushes are best. For curling, the smaller the cylinder of the brush, the tighter the curl. If you have baby-fine hair or hair strands which are very short as a result of breakage or chemical processing, you should use a small round brush and a hair-dryer and blend them in with the rest of the hair. For straightening, smaller brushes – 5–7.5cm in diameter – are suitable for shorter styles, while brushes with a larger diameter should be used on longer hair. To speed up the drying process, try a round brush that has bristles embedded in a metal or aluminium barrel, as this will heat up when it is used with a hair-dryer and so help to set and style the hair.

EXPERT ADVICE
For those who love brushing their hair vigorously, take a tip from the experts: to ensure that you do as little damage as possible, work through the hair first with a comb to deal with any tangles, before you use your hairbrush. Always brush your hair gently, trying not to pull or twist it too much. Do not brush hair when it is wet, as it will be swollen then and susceptible to damage. Hairdressers advise not brushing your hair until it is at least 80 per cent dry. If you use a styling brush before this, you risk disrupting the moisture balance of the hair, which can then lose its natural body and movement.

UPKEEP
Brushes should be washed at regular intervals with hot, soapy water. To deal with the build-up of hairs on a brush, run your comb vertically between the rows of bristles to loosen the hairs and then ease them out with your fingers. Throw away brushes and combs with broken bristles or teeth, as these can tear and snag the hair and also scratch the scalp.

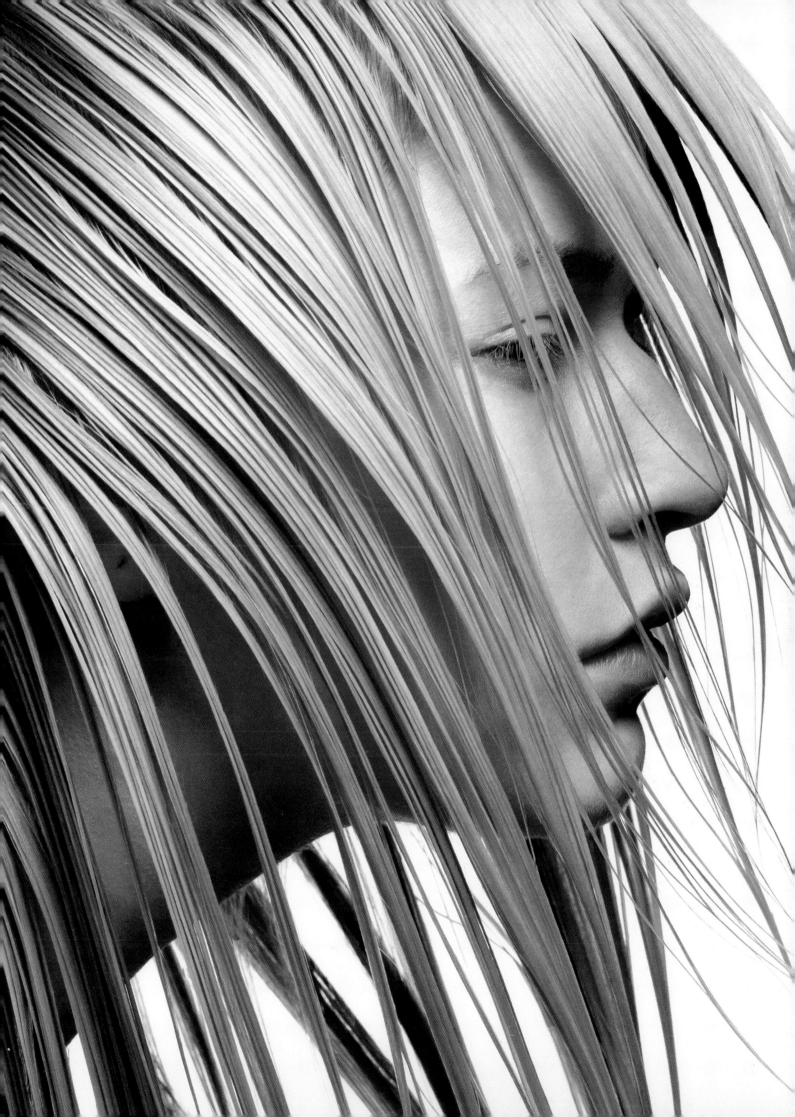

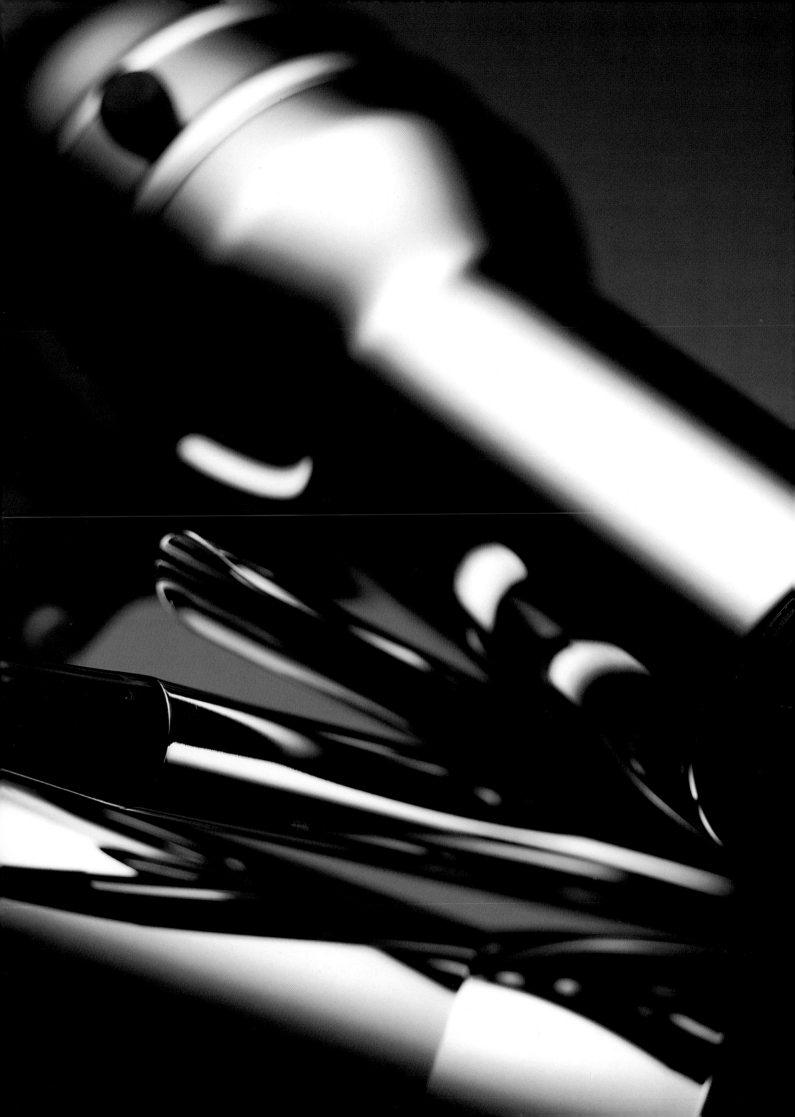

STYLING APPLIANCES

Whatever style you might want to achieve is now possible with the help of the latest heated appliances. The only drawback is that heat can damage the hair, but you can always overcome this by using a styling preparation with in-built heat protectors.

HAIR-DRYER Look for a hair-dryer with at least two speeds and three settings, cool, medium and hot. The heat from a hair-dryer can reach 60 degrees C, which is as hot as an oven. Dry your hair on the cold setting and use the warmer setting only at the end for styling the hair. Look for a 1,600+ watt dryer. Hair-dryers last on average between 200 and 300 hours of drying time. Never use a dryer without the filter in place, otherwise hair strands can get trapped in the mechanism – with disastrous results. Clean the filter regularly, as a blocked filter will cause the dryer to overheat. You should never wrap the dryer's cord tightly around it. If you have curly or permed hair, use a diffuser – a plastic or cloth attachment that fits on the end of the nozzle of the dryer – while blow-drying. This will gently spread the airflow over your hair without disturbing the curl. For the best results, switch back and forth between the low and medium settings, while cupping the hair in the palm of the hand.

TONGS These are a great device for creating curls at high speed. Choose tongs according to the type of curl you want to create, remembering that the diameter of the tongs will dictate the size of the curl. If you want to see movement right up to the roots, place a comb next to the scalp before you wind the tongs up the hair shaft to the roots. This will form a barrier to protect against burning the scalp. To clean the tongs, you should wipe with a damp cloth or alternatively use a little methylated spirit.

HOT BRUSHES These are easier to use than tongs and can create curls, tame unruly fringes or flip the ends of the hair up or under. Don't use gel or mousse when heat-styling; instead use heat-activated styling lotions and sprays, as these will hold the shape of curls without making the hair sticky or frizzy. Use hot brushes and air stylers only on dry hair. Wind the hair around the brush, working from the ends up, leave for a few seconds to let the heat penetrate the hair and then unwind. You should pin this hair in place while shaping the rest of your hair.

HEATED ROLLERS You can set your hair in ten minutes with heated rollers, which form the foundation of many styles and are a simple way to restyle the hair. The secret is to remove the rollers when they have cooled down and the hair is completely cool, otherwise the movement created will drop. Heated rollers make dealing with unruly fringes and bed-head hair quick and easy, but you should never use them on wet hair.

CRIMPERS If you want to create ripples or waves in the hair, you could try using crimpers. They often come with a range of interchangeable attachments to help you achieve different waves or straighten the hair. Use only on dry hair and avoid altogether if you have bleached hair, as the high levels of heat generated will dry the hair and this could result in breakages.

STRAIGHTENING IRONS Using a high dose of heat, these literally flatten the hair, so apply styling spray first to reduce heat damage. Use only intermittently, and never on wet, damp or bleached hair. Cordless versions are now available which makes straightening easy when you are on the move.

CUTTING EDGE

If you're planning a drastic change or want to use your hairstyle to make the most of your features, talk to your hairdresser first so as to get a good understanding of what can be achieved. There are always ways to disguise any features that you dislike.

FRINGE BENEFITS
If you have a high, a low or an uneven hairline, disguise the fact with a fringe. To draw attention away from thinning hair around the hairline, opt for a fringe which is tapered down the temples. The longer the fringe, the wider the face will appear. A round face needs a short fringe to elongate it. Wide, broad fringes can make the eyes appear larger, but can also make the face look wider. If you have a high forehead, disguise it with a longer fringe, and if you have a low forehead, choose a style with a wispy rather than a full fringe.

ROUND FACE
To flatter a round face, find a style to add height at the crown and retain overall length to elongate the face. Styles that are feathered or razor-cut at the sides soften the look and narrow the face. Shorter fringes with a blunt finish look good. Avoid bobs, flat, sleek and curly styles, hair scraped back and centre partings, as they accentuate the face's shape.

SQUARE FACE
Soften an angular face and strong jawline with a feminine cut. Opt for longer styles with casual layers or curls, a fringe which skims the top of the eyebrows to balance the proportions of the face, or a side parting. Avoid sharp, jaw-length cuts, square, heavy fringes or styles that are cropped into the nape of the neck. Remember that symmetrical and geometric shapes will only emphasize the face's shape.

LONG FACE
To balance a long face, experiment with a fringe which is cut wide into the sides of the face to give the illusion of width at the temples, and opt for a chin-length cut which will add width around the lower face. You should avoid long, straight styles, one-length cuts and styles without fringes, as these will make the shape of your face more pronounced.

OVAL FACE
This face shape is easy for hairdressers to work with because almost all hairstyles will look good with it. Oval faces do have a tendency to be wider at the forehead; if you feel this is too apparent, you could always opt for a fringe.

HEART-SHAPED FACE
Find a style which will add height at the crown and width around the jawline and chin. Feminine cuts are always the most flattering option for this shape of face. Avoid a centre parting, as this will emphasize the point of the chin. You could try a high, off-centre parting instead.

JAWLINE
Hairdressers maintain that the distance and angle between your chin and your earlobe should determine the length of your hair. If the distance is short and you have a good jawline, any length of hair will suit your face. If, however, you have a long, sloping jawline, you should really avoid very short hair styles and scraping the hair severely back from the face.

IRREGULAR FEATURES
If you have a very pointed chin, you should choose a hairstyle which adds width at the jawline to draw attention away from it. If your chin is receding, you can always make the fact less obvious by wearing your hair so the ends skim the sides of your chin. Slim down a broad neck by tucking your hair behind your ears and leaving it to softly fall around the neck. If you have a prominent nose, a soft and feminine style will be the most flattering.

CUTTING TECHNIQUES
If your hair is fine and flyaway, opt for a short layered cut which is easy to manage and will create the illusion of body. For the best results, different lengths of layers should be incorporated into the hair. If your hair is thick and frizzy, which makes it hard to handle, avoid extreme layering. Opt instead for graduated layers around the base of your hair which will help weigh the hair down and add softness.

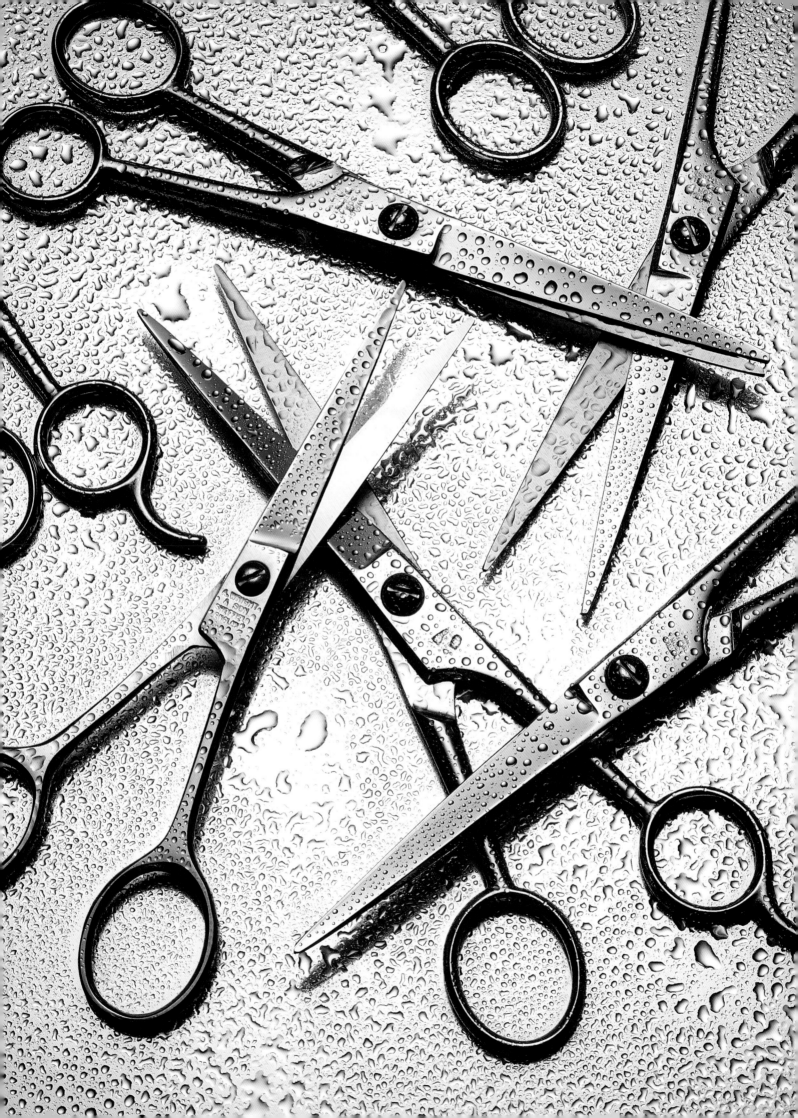

HAIRSOLUTIONS

REGULAR CUTS
It is advisable to have hair trimmed every six weeks. This helps maintain the overall condition but will not make the hair grow any quicker, contrary to popular belief. Investing in a good haircut will always pay off – as your hair grows, the style will continue to look good. Have an in-depth conversation with your hairdresser before deciding on any cut or restyle.

SPLIT ENDS
Slathering on different hair-care preparations will never repair split ends. The only way to get rid of them is to have your hair cut, but regular trims can help prevent the problem. If your hair is prone to splitting at the ends, taking a multi-vitamin supplement will strengthen it. To temporarily seal split ends, massage with moisturizer or slick with wax, serum or Vaseline.

PRODUCT OVERKILL
If you are over-using gels, mousses and sprays, your hair can end up looking dull and lifeless and may require a stripping shampoo to remove any residues, which can then play havoc with its overall condition. If you've been heavy-handed with styling preparations, brush your hair, add shampoo to it dry, massage it in and then rinse out.

WORKING OVERTIME
A creamy hair mask will double as a styling aid: mix equal amounts of the treatment mask and hair gel in the palms of the hands, apply to damp hair and mould the hair into shape. This will create a wet-look finish which will help condition the hair. When you finally rinse your hair at the end of the day, you will have glossy, healthy tresses.

follow these simple steps for healthy hair

CONDITION TIP
Leaving conditioners on for more than the time specified will not boost their effectiveness. Most conditioners only coat the hair, so they will be as effective after one minute as after fifteen. However, oil or panthenol-based deep-conditioning treatments do penetrate the hair shaft, which is why they need to be left on longer for maximum benefits.

GRIP-PROOF
Shampoos and conditioners which come in glass bottles can be a potential hazard, slipping through wet, soapy hands while you are in the bath or shower. To avoid the problem, try wrapping a couple of rubber bands round the bottles to make it easier to keep your grip. Alternatively, to be really safe, you could always just decant the contents into plastic bottles.

HEAT CHECK
If you have greasy hair, always use hair-dryers on cooler settings, as the hot air currents can activate the oil-producing glands and step up sebum production. Using a hair-dryer on a cool setting will also benefit the scalp, since unnecessary heat will make the scalp perspire fifteen minutes after drying, which will cause your hairstyle to drop and lose its shape.

GEL REVIVER
If you've slicked your hair back with gel and it starts to lose its shape and definition, you shouldn't add more product, as this could overload the hair, making it look dull and lifeless. Take a tip from the experts: wet your fingertips and run them through your hair to resculpt and revitalize it. Alternatively, brush the hair to remove the gel and restart from scratch.

BEAUTY INTELLIGENCE

1 Tip your head upside-down when brushing to speed blood flow to the scalp and also to get at the stronger, more protected hair usually hidden underneath.

2 You should never try to dress freshly washed hair. The natural oils present in unwashed hair will make it much easier to control, helping with your styling.

3 Try to hold your hair-dryer above and behind your head, like your hairdresser will normally do. The hot air will then flow down the hair shaft and over the cuticles.

4 Scrunch equal amounts of hair gel and serum into curls that are frizzy and fluffy. Serum will stop the gel stiffening as it dries, stop curls frizzing and boost shine.

5 You shouldn't try running a comb through curled hair but should use your fingers to break up the curls instead, otherwise you'll end up with a frizzy mess.

6 To give dull, lifeless-looking hair high-speed shine, add serum to the mid-lengths and run a large make-up brush gently down the hair shaft to smooth the cuticles.

7 If you have sensitive eyes, you should use baby shampoo. This will not cause any irritation if you get splashed, even when you're rinsing your hair, as it's so mild.

8 Hair serum, which can be used to protect and to polish the tresses, can also be smoothed on to bare legs in the summer to give skin a more flattering finish.

9 You can massage styling wax into nail cuticles to hydrate and protect them. Gently heat the wax with a hair-dryer first, as it will be easier to apply when soft.

10 Whatever the temptations, do try not to keep touching your hair once it has been styled; otherwise, it can lose its shape and body, and become greasy.

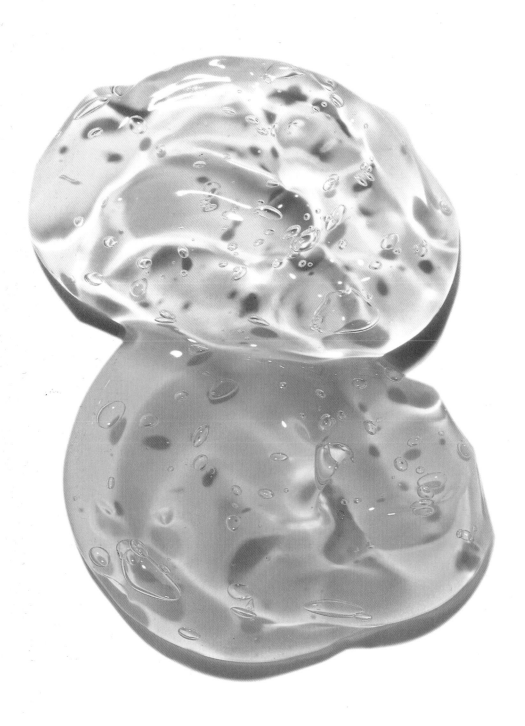

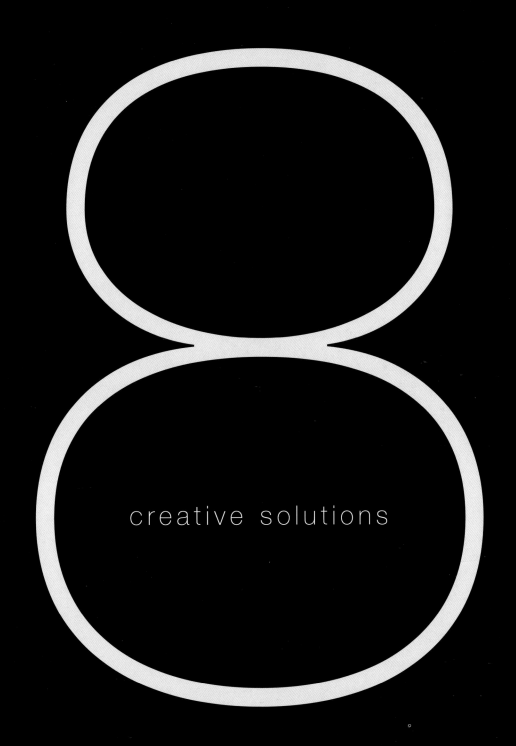

creative solutions

Hair-styling can be achieved at high speed with minimum fuss as long as you know how. Whether you want to create curls, wear your hair up or let it hang loose, the aim is to look sexy, modern and natural. Over-worked hair can seem artificial and dated. Any hairstyle should give the impression that you created it effortlessly in a few minutes.

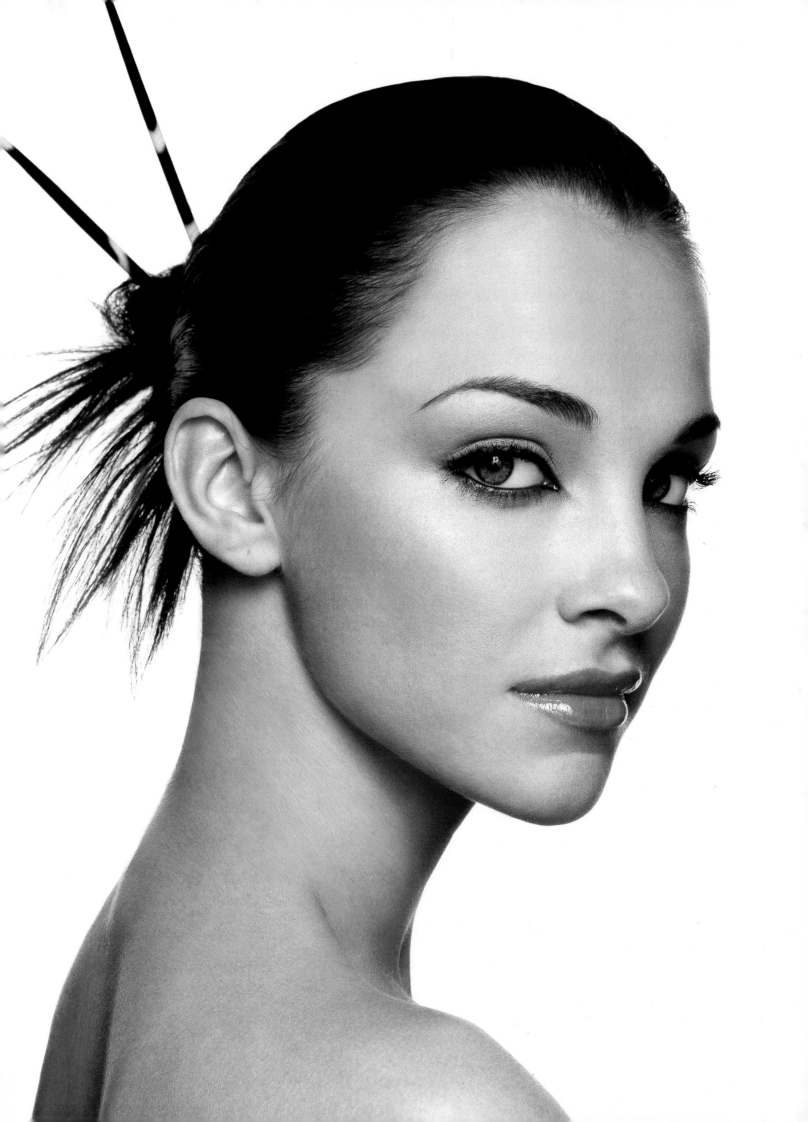

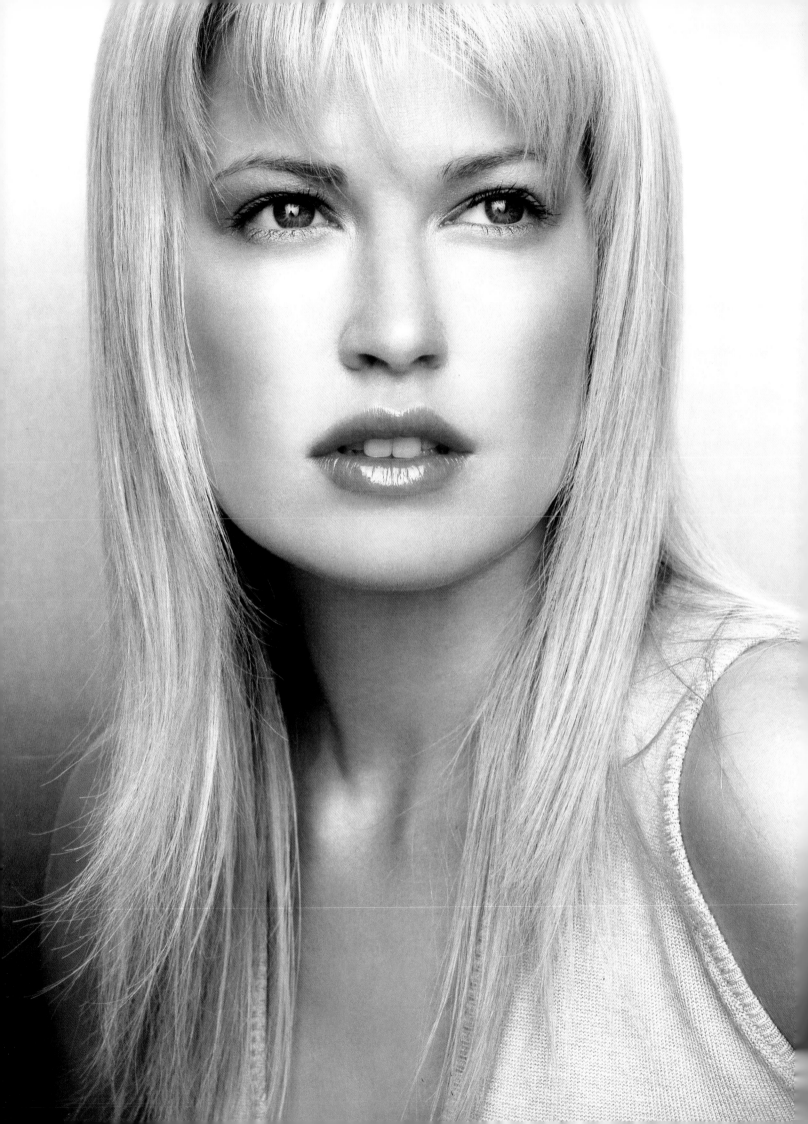

BLOW DRYING

PREP WORK Before blow-drying, use a wide-toothed comb to remove all tangles. Apply a heat-styling aid to protect the hair and comb through in the direction and shape of the finished style. Start off rough-drying the hair all over and then blow-dry the under sections, making sure that each one is completely dry before moving on to the next, and gradually work up the head. Hot hair can feel damp, so give your hair a cool blast of air before you decide whether it is really dry or not.

STYLING ADVICE Never attempt to style your hair when it is wet. Instead, rough-dry it with a hair-dryer using your hands until it is 50–60 per cent dry if curly and 80 per cent if straight. The more styling your hair needs, the damper it should be. To speed up this initial drying stage, tip your head upside-down and use your hair-dryer to remove any excess moisture.

DRYING TECHNIQUES You should always move the dryer as you are working on the hair, even when you are concentrating on one particular section. Either work in small rotating motions or gently shake the dryer, as the heat will dry the hair out and can burn the scalp if you are drying the roots.

HEAT CONTROL Do not use a dryer on the hottest setting when you are working on the roots, as this can irritate and burn the scalp, and make the hair greasy. It will also flatten the hair. Moderate heat (or slightly hotter for frizzy or thick hair) will help create volume. If your hair is fine, always work with the dryer on a cool to moderate setting to stop it being dried out.

KEEP COOL If you are using a brush while blow-drying to curl or style your hair, you should allow each section of hair to cool before removing the brush, otherwise the movement you have created might drop. Alternatively, before removing the brush, blast the hair with the dryer on a cool setting to finish.

COWLICKS A cowlick is a small area of hair which sticks up around the hairline and does not grow in the same direction as the rest of the hair. To tame it, you will need to anchor the hair with a round brush in the opposite direction to usual and blow-dry, holding the brush firmly in place. If you then blow-dry in the other direction, this should straighten the cowlick out.

AIR FLOW Always aim the air flow of your hair-dryer down the hair shaft, to ensure that the cuticles lie flat and the hair looks shiny (if you point the air flow up the hair shaft, it will dishevel the cuticles and the hair will look dull and lifeless). To make this task easier and to give yourself greater control of where the heat is going, hold the nozzle instead of the handle of the dryer in your hand and work from the roots to the ends.

LIMITED TIME If you are pushed for time, start blow-drying the hair around your face first, as these are the bits on show, and then work on the top sections. If time does not permit, leave the under sections to dry naturally. Alternatively, comb wet hair into shape and then leave; when nearly dry, get to work with your hair-dryer and a styling brush to finish off.

TWISTER

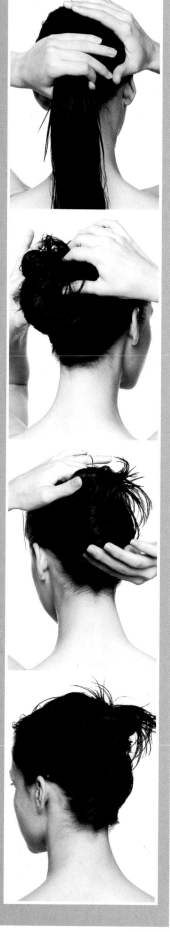

1. You don't need to be an expert to master this style. If you arm yourself with a comb and hair grips, you can twist your hair up into an interesting shape in seconds. Comb through and scrape all the hair back to the nape of the neck, as if creating a ponytail. Instead of securing with a band, twist the hair until it is taut and then twist up the head.

2. Secure in place with randomly placed pins where needed, but make sure the pins are not visible. If you have problems seeing what you are doing, look into a wall mirror and then inspect your work with a hand-held mirror, holding it behind you.

3. If you find that stray hairs have dropped from your original section of hair, use the pointed tail end of the comb and gently scrape them back in, securing with extra pins.

4. This is a great style for you to create when your hair is still wet, because it will then dry in place. It will also give the hair interesting movement and body when you take the pins out and unravel your hair.

PONYTAIL

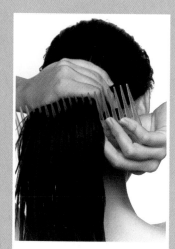

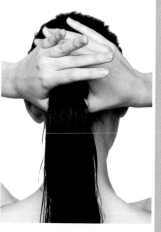

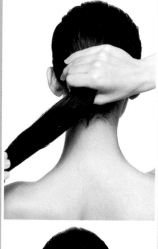

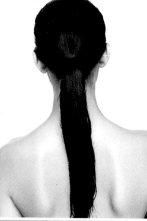

1. Anyone can achieve this look in four simple steps. It is a great way to disguise greasy-looking hair: simply add a small amount of gel and then continue. Or you can work without using any styling preparations at all. Start by combing the hair to make sure that it is completely tangle-free.

2. Comb hair back towards the nape of the neck. Ensure that the hair is tightly pulled back by running the hands through. This will tame unruly hairs and reduce static that may have occurred while combing.

3. Do not secure with a rubber band as they can snag and tear the hair and are difficult to remove. Look for special bands that are either fabric-covered or designed not to rip hair.

4. Once in place, roughly divide your ponytail into two parts and draw them out vertically to tighten the fastening. Comb through again for a sleek finish. For added interest, you could always curl the ends of your hair or add extra shine by smoothing serum on to the hair that is scraped back into the ponytail.

CURLS

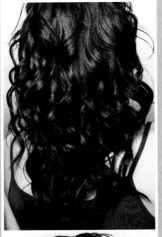

1. If you have a natural wave to your hair it will be easy to curl, whereas straight hair will need more work. Curl hair by setting with rollers (using heated rollers on dry hair or Velcro rollers on damp hair). The type of curl created will be determined by the size of rollers used: the smaller the rollers, the tighter the curl. Large rollers will create rough and tumble, loose curls. Spray with a sculpting or setting lotion before using rollers.

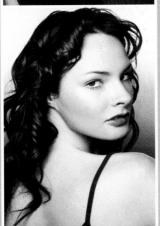

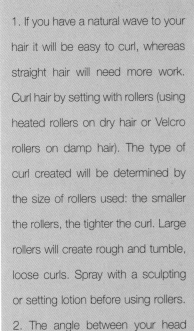

2. The angle between your head and the position of your hair before you roll it will determine the amount of root lift. So, if hair is wound round the roller at a 90-degree angle it will create maximum root lift, while 45 degrees will give minimum root lift.

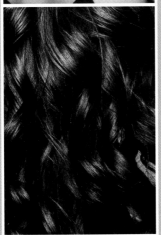

3. Always wind hair round the roller from the ends up. Use Velcro rollers so you do not need to secure with pins and so don't mark the hair.

4. Do not remove rollers until hair is completely dry, or the movement will simply drop out. To dress curls, do not comb them through, using your fingers to separate them instead.

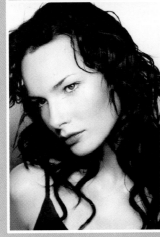

SLICK

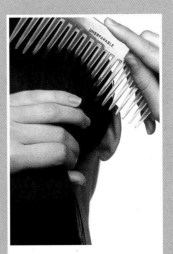

1. Slicking it back is one of the simplest and quickest ways to style the hair. Create either a high-shine, slick finish or a more textured variation. You can slick wet or dry hair back. For a more natural-looking finish, use a minimal amount of hair mousse or gel and gently run a wide-toothed comb through dry or damp hair; for a sleeker finish, smooth wax or pomade on to the hair and then comb in place. If you do not have gel, mousse or wax to hand, use an oil-based moisturizer to slick hair back. It will not brush out, so you will need to wash it out.

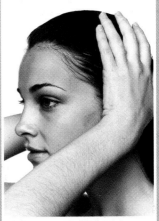

2. Carefully work the comb through the hair to distribute the product evenly and then shape into the desired style. A wide-toothed comb will create an interesting finish.

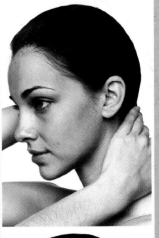

3. After combing, run the hands through to tame any stray hairs and ensure a smooth finish. To keep in place, apply a fine mist of hairspray.

4. If you have long hair you can slick it back and then go on to either secure it in a ponytail or pin it up.

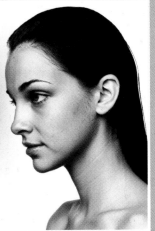

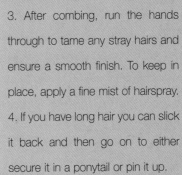

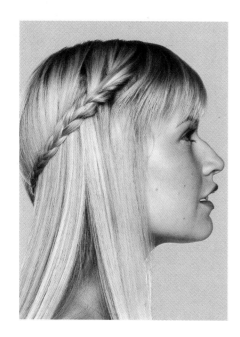

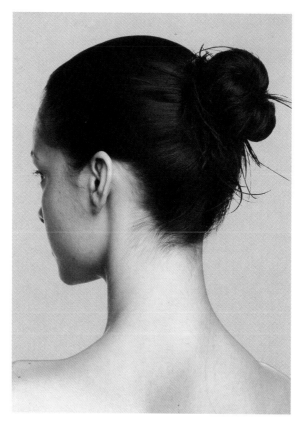

2

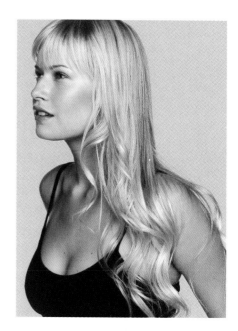

3

DROP CURLS

If you have shoulder-length or longer hair which is straight or has a natural wave, you can create an interesting finish by curling the mid-lengths (just below the ears) and ends. Start at the front with 2.5cm-wide sections of hair and wrap them around heated tongs, working from the mid-lengths to the ends. Clasp hair in tongs for thirty to sixty seconds, depending on your hair type: fine hair will absorb heat more quickly. Unravel and then move on to the next section. If you're using heated rollers, follow the same procedure but wind hair from the ends up the hair shaft until you reach the tops of the ears. Secure in place and move on to the next section.

1

BRAID

If you are looking for a variation on normal plaits, you can braid simply the front section of your hair at each side of the temple and then scrape these back and let the rest of the hair hang straight down. This is a great way to add interest to a one-length style. If you are bored with the traditional three-strand plait and want to try something different, use just two sections of hair and weave them together. When you get to the ends of the hair, secure the braids with a band.

TOPKNOT

Ensure hair is tangle-free, then comb it towards the crown of the head and scrape into a high ponytail. Secure with a ponytail tie, then wrap the hair in a circular motion round the tie in a bun shape. Secure with hair grips or bobby pins. For a modern finish, splay the ends out and mould into an interesting shape, then fix with a light hairspray. You could reposition the bun at the nape of the neck or the middle of the back of the head.

six secrets for easy ways with hair-styling

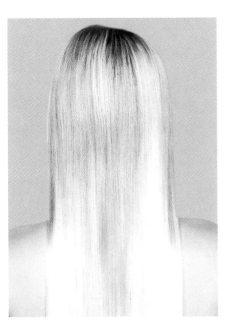

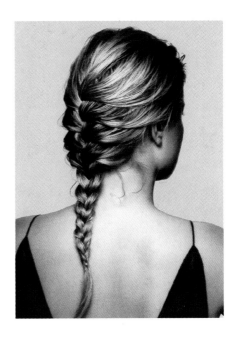

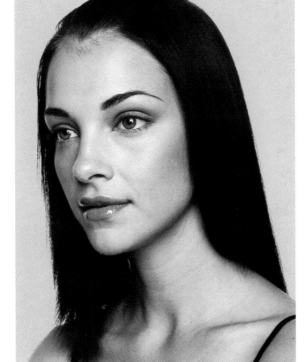

4

STRAIGHT

To blow-dry your hair dead straight, first apply mousse, then comb it through and partially rough-dry the hair. Take a 2.5cm section across the hair at the nape of the neck with a comb and pin the rest of the hair out of the way. Using a round brush, dry this section. For the best results, glide the brush from roots to ends and direct the air flow from the hair-dryer down the hair shaft, following the brush as you work. Make sure that each section is completely dry before you move on to the next one. Gradually proceed up the head, working in 2.5cm sections. After drying, smooth on a small amount of serum to give the hair a polished finish.

5

SCRAPE BACK

Ideal for one-length styles, longer hair with layers or if you are growing a fringe out. The secret is to ensure that the hair is absolutely straight and ultra-shiny. If you're not expert at blow-drying your hair straight, get to work with heated straightening irons. Once hair is straight, comb it off the face and make two partings (using the centre of each iris as a guide) back to the crown. Hold this section at a 90-degree angle to the head, scrape a hair comb the same width in and push back, so it grips the hair, taking it off the face. Push back until the comb feels secure.

6

PLAIT

To successfully plait the hair, comb through to remove tangles and then divide into three equal sections. Weave the left section over the middle section, then weave the right section over the middle section, repeating the process until you reach the end of the hair. Secure with a band. Once you have finished, you can spritz the hair with a fine mist of hairspray to keep it in place. If you feel the total look is too neat, simply ease out a few strands of hair around the front. If you pull too much out by mistake, you don't need to start again from scratch. Using small pins, scoop hair back into the plait and secure in place.

STYLINGWORK

STYLE SAVERS
When you are travelling, it's always possible to get more mileage from your hair-styling appliances. When you are packing, wrap your necklaces around a hair roller and secure in place with a hair elastic. This will ensure that chains do not tangle and get knotted. Also, hair-dyers can be used to dry lingerie and any other small items of clothing after washing.

MIRROR IMAGE
If you have a symmetrically shaped hairstyle, you should alternate the hand in which you hold the dryer in order to ensure that both sides of the hair look the same. Once you have mastered the knack and it comes naturally, you will be blow-drying like a professional. As a side effect, this is a good way to tone the muscles on both arms and hands.

SATIN SLIP
If you always wake up with bed-head hair, you could try changing your pillowcase. Satin pillowcases allow the hair to slide across the pillow gently as you move in your sleep, whereas cotton causes friction and disrupts the hair. Using a satin pillowcase also means that you will not end up with crease marks on your face if you tend to sleep nuzzled into the pillow.

EASY CURLS
To curl hair with a natural wave, take random 5–7.5cm sections of damp hair, twist tightly and literally scrunch up into small balls and secure in place. Leave to dry naturally, only unravelling when the hair is completely dry. To finish, do not comb through but tip your head upside-down and use your fingers to break up the curl and enhance the movement created.

simple steps to successful hair-styling

ROOT LIFT

A foolproof way that is guaranteed to achieve root lift which will not drop shortly afterwards is to work through the roots with a vent brush. While you are blow-drying your hair, lift individual sections as you go. You will also find that tipping your head upside-down or leaning your head to one side as you blow-dry has the effect of maximizing the hair's volume.

FLYAWAY HAIR

If you have a problem with static, flyaway hair, you could always try using an anti-static clothes spray. You should never apply this directly to the hair, but can spray a small amount on to a comb or hairbrush and then gently run it through the hair. However, you should go lightly at this stage, as over-zealous combing or brushing is likely to result in more static.

STEAM STYLE

When you run a bath, close the bathroom door so the steam from the water doesn't evaporate, then spray your hair with setting lotion and put rollers in before getting into the bath. The steam will help set the curls. Remove the rollers when your hair is completely dry and run your fingers through the hair to break up the curls and to add definition.

THICKENING TREAT

If you have baby-fine blonde hair and want to make it look fuller and also appear white blonde, hairdressers recommend spraying the hair with dry shampoo. This will add body and make the hair easier to manage. Just remember, less is more, so try to be as light-handed as possible during application. To remove, you can simply brush the hair.

157

BEAUTY INTELLIGENCE

If you have Afro hair and no styling products, try jojoba oil instead. Similar in structure to the hair's own oil, it will hydrate, condition and help with shine.

As we age, it is sometimes more flattering to opt for a hairstyle with greater volume and body, so avoid styles that are too sleek or worn flat against the head.

After using hairspray, try not to brush your hair, otherwise you will remove all the product you have just added. Instead run a comb gently through your hair.

Take a bottle of conditioner to the beach to shield the hair from UV rays. The heat intensifies the product's activity, so even after a day in the sun hair will not suffer.

If your hair looks flat a few hours after styling, give it a boost by tipping the head down and running a brush through it to trap air in, creating instant volume.

As we age, hair becomes fragile and susceptible to damage, so use a hairbrush with soft bristles and keep chemical processing and heat-styling to a minimum.

Don't be fooled into thinking big hair and loads of make-up mean glamour. The secret is always to choose styles that are simple, so creating an understated look.

To give hair movement and body, wrap it up when wet and leave to dry. This creates gentle rather than rigid-looking waves and doesn't require any rollers.

To add interesting texture to dry hair without it looking greasy or overloaded with product, you could work through a small amount of leave-in conditioner.

If you snag your tights, use a little hairspray to stop the ladder from running. Do not be heavy-handed, though, or your tights might end up stuck to your legs.

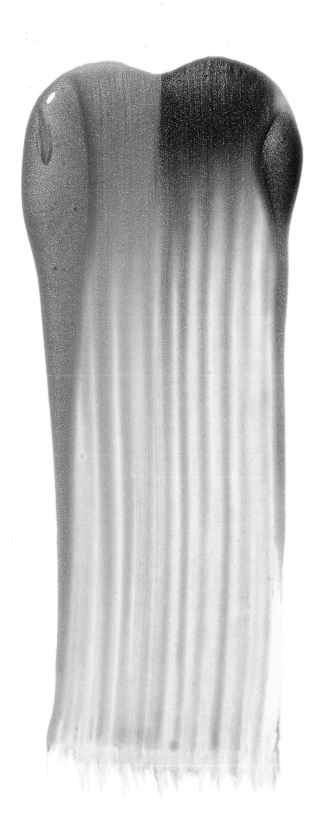

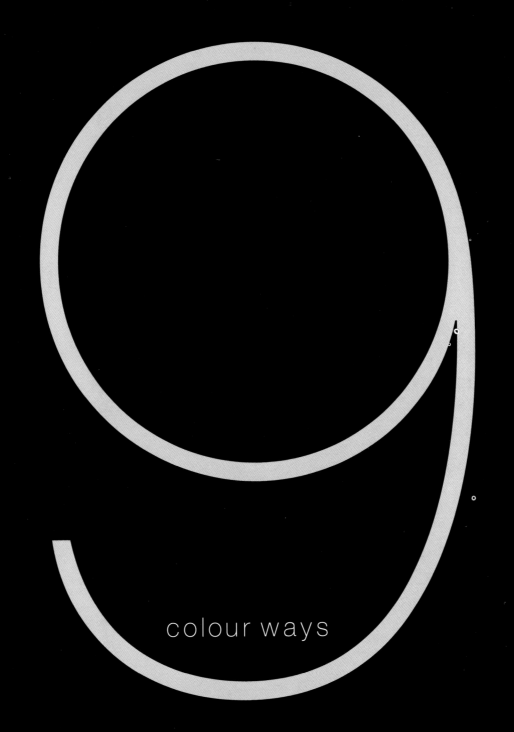

colour ways

Whether you go for bold red, rich brown or glossy blonde, hair colour can make a great impact on the way you look and feel. The new generation of colorants are enriched with conditioning ingredients, so if you want a drastic change or just subtle enhancement, you can achieve results which are now no longer detrimental to the overall health of your hair.

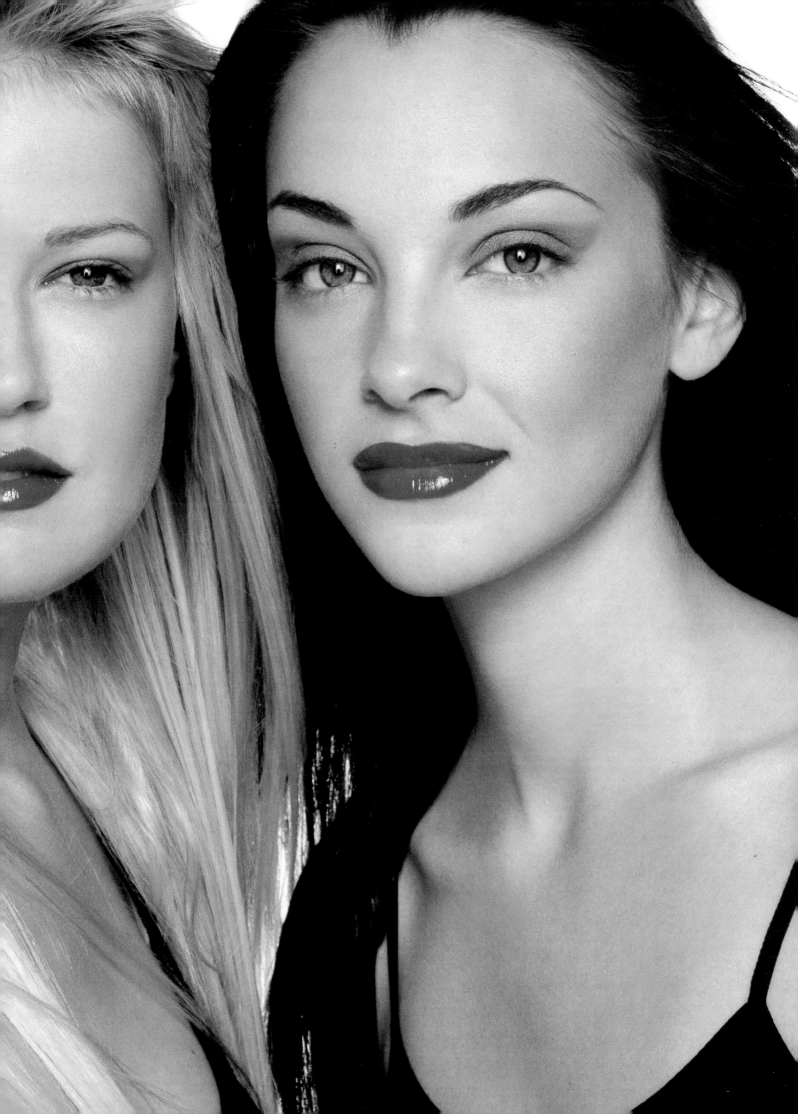

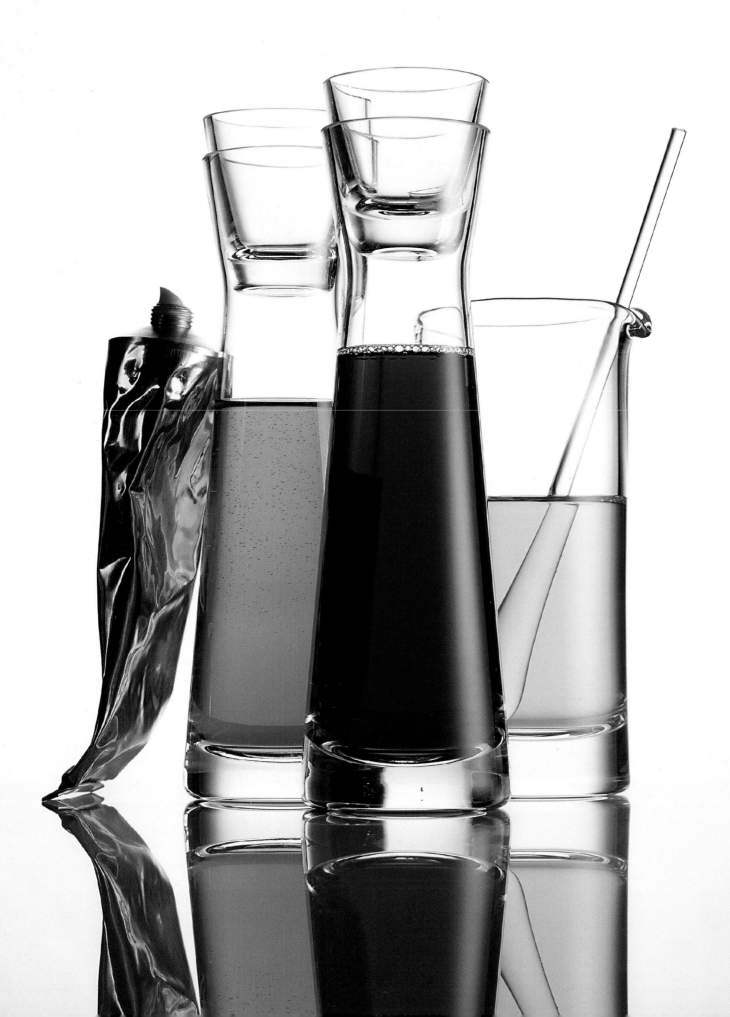

HAIR COLOUR

TEMPORARY COLOURS Mousse, shampoo, setting lotions, hairsprays and rinses coat the cuticles, forming a film of temporary colour in an instant which will wash out when the hair is shampooed. They are designed for minor changes to darken the tone of or intensify your natural colour but unless specified do not have the ability to lighten the hair or conceal grey hair. You will need to seek advice before using on hair which is already colour-treated or permed. Ash-blonde and silver shades are useful to brighten grey or white hair which looks yellow or dingy from cigarette smoke or pollution build-up.

SEMI-PERMANENTS Like temporary colorants, semi-permanents coat the hair shaft with colour pigments, but they will last between five and seven washes, depending on how porous the hair is. If your hair is dry and damaged, it will absorb some of the colour pigments, so the colour will wash out less easily. Semi-permanent colours will not turn dark hair blonde but are ideal for enhancing your natural colour, adding shine and concealing grey (just be wary of red tones), and are a great way to experiment without being stuck with the results for too long. This type of colorant should be applied to damp hair, which is then shampooed once the colour has developed.

TONE-ON-TONE These are longer-lasting versions of semi-permanent colour which gradually fade between twelve and twenty washes. They penetrate the hair shaft slightly (so there can be signs of regrowth at the roots) and have more holding power, but they cannot lighten the hair. They are recommended for enhancing natural hair colour, making hair a deeper colour or covering hair that is up to 60 per cent grey.

PERMANENT COLOUR This type of colorant, which won't wash out, is available in three forms. First, there is henna, a natural long-lasting dye that can be removed only by cutting, which literally stains the hair. Then there are metallic dyes, also known as colour restorers, which are sold as 'banish grey hair' colorants. They deposit metallic dyes and salts from various metals, such as silver, cobalt, copper and magnesium, on the hair shaft which gradually darken. Finally, there are chemical dyes or tints, which are the most commonly used form of permanent colour and come in the widest range of colours. They work by opening up the cuticles so the colour pigments enter the cortex. After the colour has developed, the cuticles are closed, thus trapping in the colour pigments permanently. This type of treatment will allow you to tint your hair up to four shades lighter than your natural colour. The only drawback with permanent tints is that, as the hair grows, the roots will need retouching – usually every six to eight weeks.

BLEACHING If you want all your hair lightened or are looking for results that cannot be achieved with high-lift tint, you can bleach your hair. The strong alkaline solution used in bleaching raises the cuticles and the bleach will lighten the hair's natural pigments. Each hair goes through a colour change from black to dark brown, red brown, golden brown, golden blonde and light blonde as the bleaching agents lighten the pigments. Rinsing stops the process at the shade you require. Unless you really know what you are doing, you should leave the job to the experts, as colour changes can be unpredictable. Due to the harsh chemical processing involved, hair can break easily and the product can burn the scalp if left on too long. If your scalp is prone to sensitivity, bleaching is not to be recommended. As it is the harshest of the colour processes, you should follow a conditioning and restructuring after-care programme. Semi-permanent colours can be applied to bleached hair to add colour and help improve condition.

HIGHLIGHTS AND LOWLIGHTS By using bleach or tint to highlight your hair, you can weave in up to three different tones of colour to create an effect similar to sun-kissed lightening. Alternatively, you can add contrasting shades to your natural colour for a more striking effect. Lowlights can introduce deeper glints to the hair, darkening it in places or adding intensely toned colours such as copper, gold and red, which look great on dark blonde and brown hair. As your hair grows, the roots will need retouching, probably after six or eight weeks.

COLOUR CHOICE

Hair colour, like make-up, must suit your complexion. If you have a pale or ivory-coloured skin, any hair colour will look good. Women with a pink flush to their skin should avoid shades of red or golden blonde, opting for ash tones to neutralize their colouring. Those with more sallow-looking complexions should avoid yellow, gold or orange tones, going for deep reds and burgundies. Black skin will be complemented by colours similar to the natural hair colour. Those with olive skin tones should stay dark, adding richness to their hair with lowlights in red shades that range from chestnut to burgundy.

TEST RUN

If you have never coloured your hair before, always try a test patch for sensitivity before you start. Wipe a 1cm section of skin behind the ear with cotton wool soaked in surgical spirit and then dab on a little hair tint using a cotton bud. Reapply two or three times, allowing the tint to dry between each application. Don't wash the area for forty-eight hours. After this time, if there is no skin redness or itching, the product will be safe to use. Never try shading the eyebrows or tinting the eyelashes with hair colorants. Because they are not formulated for use on sensitive areas, you could suffer from adverse reactions.

ON TRIAL

If you want to see the end results before you undergo a colour change, cut off a tiny piece of hair close to the roots. Use a piece of sticky tape to hold the strands together at one end, then apply the colour mixture. Leave on for the specified time, rinse out and wait until the hair is dry, then judge the results. This is a particularly good idea if your hair has already gone through chemical processing and is coloured or permed, as the end results can be unpredictable. Alternatively, to see what different hair colours will look like against your skin, try on wigs and hairpieces in shades you are considering.

CLEAN UP

If you are not a professional applying colour at home, follow these simple steps to make the task easier. Rub Vaseline into the skin around the hairline before applying colour to act as a protective barrier and prevent staining of the skin. To remove after the colour processing, massage a small amount of cream cleanser into the Vaseline and then remove with damp cotton wool. Always wear gloves while applying colour and wrap a dark-coloured, old towel around your shoulders. If you get colour in your eyes, rinse with lots of water immediately and if irritation or reactions persist consult a GP.

DOS AND DON'TS

Never use tints, especially permanent varieties or 'anti-grey' colour restorers, over henna, as there could be an adverse chemical reaction to the metallic compounds, leaving you with a hair colour you never expected. Mix up the colour before applying and then discard after using, unless the manufacturer's instructions suggest it will be safe to use again at a later date. Always use plastic rather than metal tools when mixing colour. If you have had a perm, wait at least forty-eight hours before using a colorant. You should get your hair cut or reshaped after chemical processing, as even the healthiest hair will be porous around the ends and show damage.

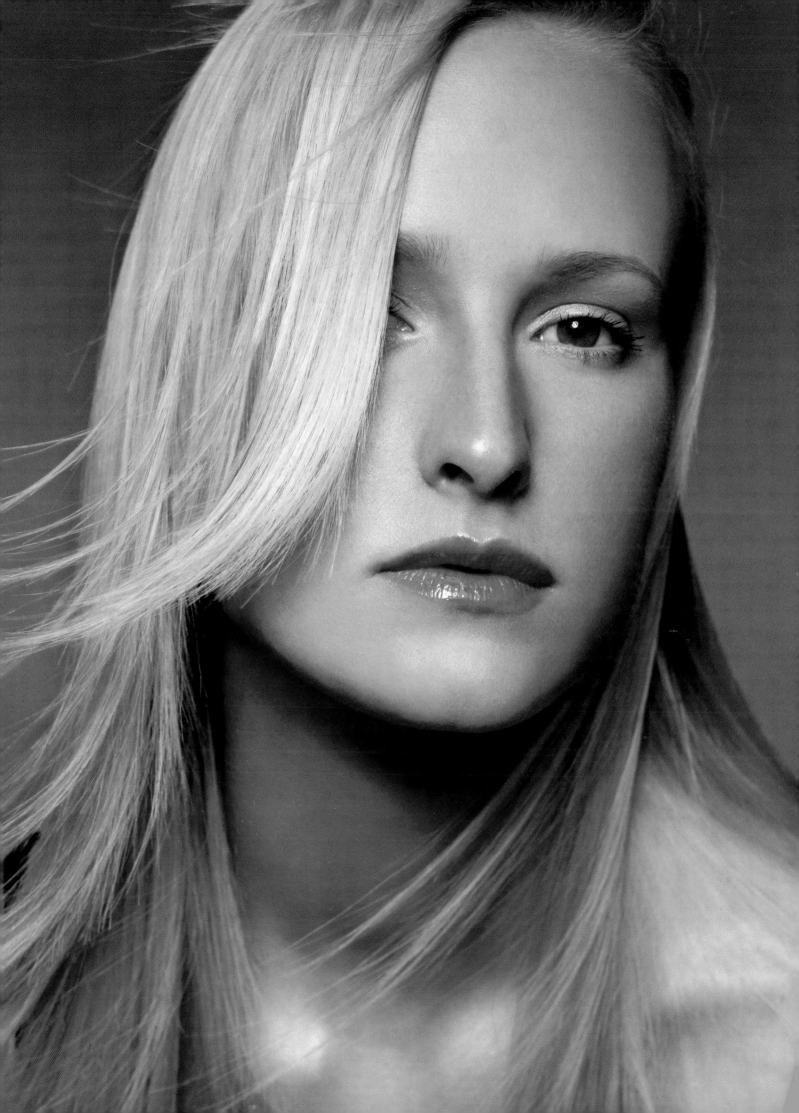

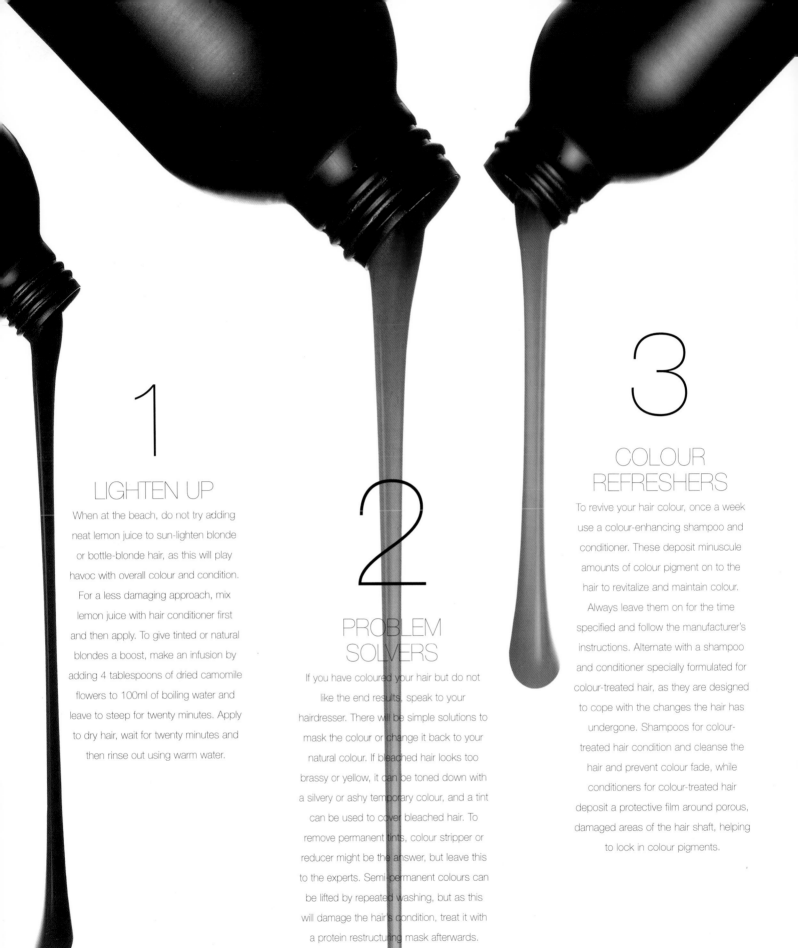

1

LIGHTEN UP

When at the beach, do not try adding
neat lemon juice to sun-lighten blonde
or bottle-blonde hair, as this will play
havoc with overall colour and condition.
For a less damaging approach, mix
lemon juice with hair conditioner first
and then apply. To give tinted or natural
blondes a boost, make an infusion by
adding 4 tablespoons of dried camomile
flowers to 100ml of boiling water and
leave to steep for twenty minutes. Apply
to dry hair, wait for twenty minutes and
then rinse out using warm water.

2

PROBLEM
SOLVERS

If you have coloured your hair but do not
like the end results, speak to your
hairdresser. There will be simple solutions to
mask the colour or change it back to your
natural colour. If bleached hair looks too
brassy or yellow, it can be toned down with
a silvery or ashy temporary colour, and a tint
can be used to cover bleached hair. To
remove permanent tints, colour stripper or
reducer might be the answer, but leave this
to the experts. Semi-permanent colours can
be lifted by repeated washing, but as this
will damage the hair's condition, treat it with
a protein restructuring mask afterwards.

3

COLOUR
REFRESHERS

To revive your hair colour, once a week
use a colour-enhancing shampoo and
conditioner. These deposit minuscule
amounts of colour pigment on to the
hair to revitalize and maintain colour.
Always leave them on for the time
specified and follow the manufacturer's
instructions. Alternate with a shampoo
and conditioner specially formulated for
colour-treated hair, as they are designed
to cope with the changes the hair has
undergone. Shampoos for colour-
treated hair condition and cleanse the
hair and prevent colour fade, while
conditioners for colour-treated hair
deposit a protective film around porous,
damaged areas of the hair shaft, helping
to lock in colour pigments.

six secrets for colour maintenance

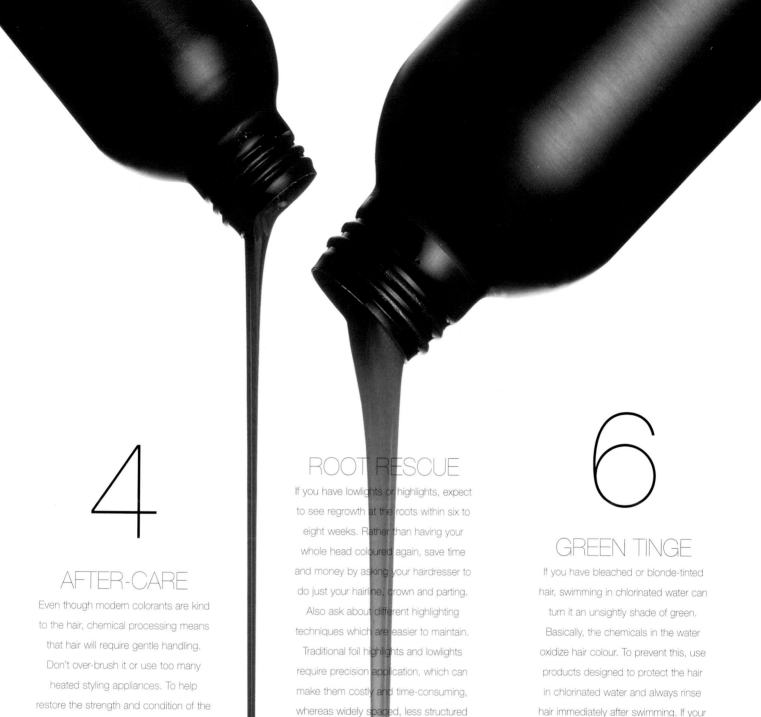

4

AFTER-CARE

Even though modern colorants are kind to the hair, chemical processing means that hair will require gentle handling. Don't over-brush it or use too many heated styling appliances. To help restore the strength and condition of the hair, use extra-nourishing conditioners, hair masks and protein restructurants. When you wash your hair, always finish off by rinsing with cold water as this will close the cuticles, ensuring that they lie flat, which helps the hair's natural resilience and also makes it look shiny.

ROOT RESCUE

If you have lowlights or highlights, expect to see regrowth at the roots within six to eight weeks. Rather than having your whole head coloured again, save time and money by asking your hairdresser to do just your hairline, crown and parting. Also ask about different highlighting techniques which are easier to maintain. Traditional foil highlights and lowlights require precision application, which can make them costly and time-consuming, whereas widely spaced, less structured slices of colour are much easier to retouch or change.

5

6

GREEN TINGE

If you have bleached or blonde-tinted hair, swimming in chlorinated water can turn it an unsightly shade of green. Basically, the chemicals in the water oxidize hair colour. To prevent this, use products designed to protect the hair in chlorinated water and always rinse hair immediately after swimming. If your hair does have a green tinge, either book in to see your hairdresser or follow this correcting method: pour tomato juice on to the hair, massage it in, leave for a couple of minutes and then rinse out. The tomato juice will neutralize the green colour and help restore natural, and not so natural, blondes to their former glory.

COLOURADVICE

HENNA HELP

Think carefully before using henna to colour your hair. It can give unpredictable results, can't be removed without cutting your hair and can't be used with other colorants as the organic minerals it contains can react disastrously with them. The only way to improve a bad henna job is by using a chemical-free semi-permanent colour, but consult your hairdresser first.

COLOUR FADE

Aim to colour your hair four to six weeks before going on holiday or heading for the sun, so it has time to rebalance before being exposed to harmful UV rays. Since sunlight works on the hair like peroxide, lifting the colour and accelerating dryness and damage, protect your hair by applying preparations that are enriched with UV filters or slick wax through.

BRUNETTE BOOST

Don't waste money on expensive products to boost hair colour. Try brewing a double espresso, leaving it to cool and then using it as an infusion for dark hair: pour over dry hair, wait thirty minutes and rinse. Alternatively, steep 2 teaspoons of walnut leaves and a teabag in warm water, leave to cool, then use as a post-shampooing rinse for dark hair.

COMING CLEAN

If you've coloured your hair at home and stained the skin, rub with a cotton-wool pad soaked with alcohol-based toner, or scrub with hot soapy water and a nailbrush. Some experts advise massaging whitening toothpaste into the skin, leaving it for five minutes and then removing with a tissue, or even working cold cigarette ash in to lift the colour.

all you need to know about colorants

NATURAL COLOUR
Certain hair colours will suit your natural colour better than others. If your hair is dark to light brown, add streaks – go dark or red; if it's black, avoid going blonde or red; if it's dark to light blonde, opt for warm shades from honey to milky brown and chestnut; if it's grey/blonde, opt for pale, cool tones; and if it's grey, avoid going red.

COLOUR PRECAUTIONS
Doubts exist about the safety of permanent and semi-permanent colorants for pregnant women, so avoid colouring methods that apply dye direct to the scalp and go instead for low- or highlights or a vegetable colour. After three months, as hormonal changes improve your hair's condition, you may decide not to use colour anyway.

COVER-UP
When melanin production stops, the hair becomes white, although this is perceived as grey. If you have up to 60 per cent grey hair, try a tone-on-tone colour, which will last up to twenty washes. If you are above 60 per cent grey, consider a permanent colour. If you are happy with your natural grey, use a colour-enhancing shampoo to bring out the silver tones.

VEGETABLE COLOURS
Made from natural extracts, vegetable colours literally stain the hair when shampooed in and will last up to six washes. They boost natural shine and revitalize dull-looking locks but will not conceal grey. If you have bleached or colour-treated hair, the results can be unpredictable; if hair is dry and damaged, the colour will remain true for longer.

BEAUTY INTELLIGENCE

After colouring do not wash hair or expose to chlorinated water or strong sunlight for forty-eight hours, as it will interfere with the results and the hair's condition.

If you have used a semi-permanent colour on your hair but you don't like the results, use a clarifying or body-building shampoo to fade colour quickly.

If you have fine hair, remember that using permenent colour can make it appear thicker, as the chemical processing involved will cause the hair shaft to swell.

Bear in mind the colour of your eyes and brows before opting for a colour change. If you've lightened your hair, use a facial bleaching kit to lift brow colour.

If you have greasy locks, the experts recommend using a hair colorant, because the chemical processes involved will change the natural porosity of your hair.

By adding highlights or lowlights you will break up the heaviness of very thick hair; they will also enhance fine hair by creating greater texture and more body.

6

7

Your choice of hair colour is vital. If the colour is too light, it can make the hair look thinner, while rich tones will reflect more light and make it look much thicker.

To brighten the complexion, add a few subtle highlights to the hair around the face. Opt for tones which warm the skin and enhance your natural hair colour.

8

9

If you have short hair, steer clear of highlights as they can result in a leopard-print effect. For the best results, try using a semi-permanent or permanent colour.

You should treat coloured hair with a hydrating mask once a week to replace lost moisture, but avoid hot-oil treatments as they tend to strip out hair colour.

10

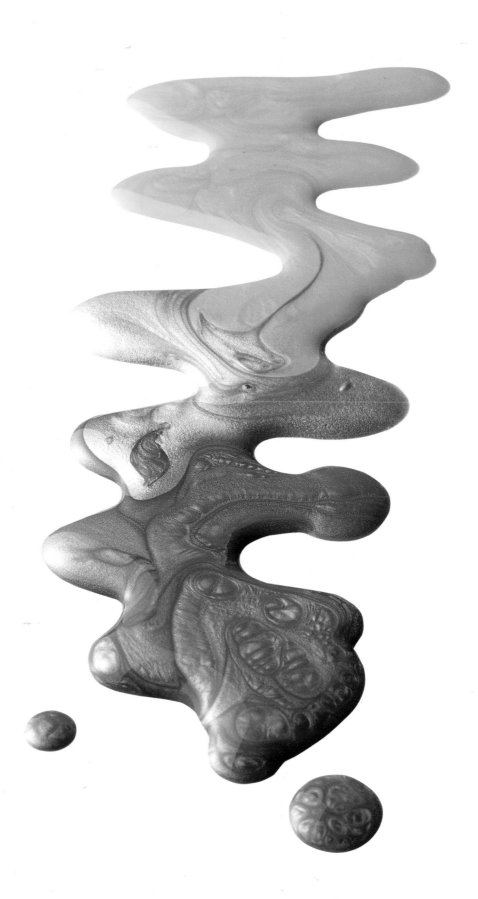

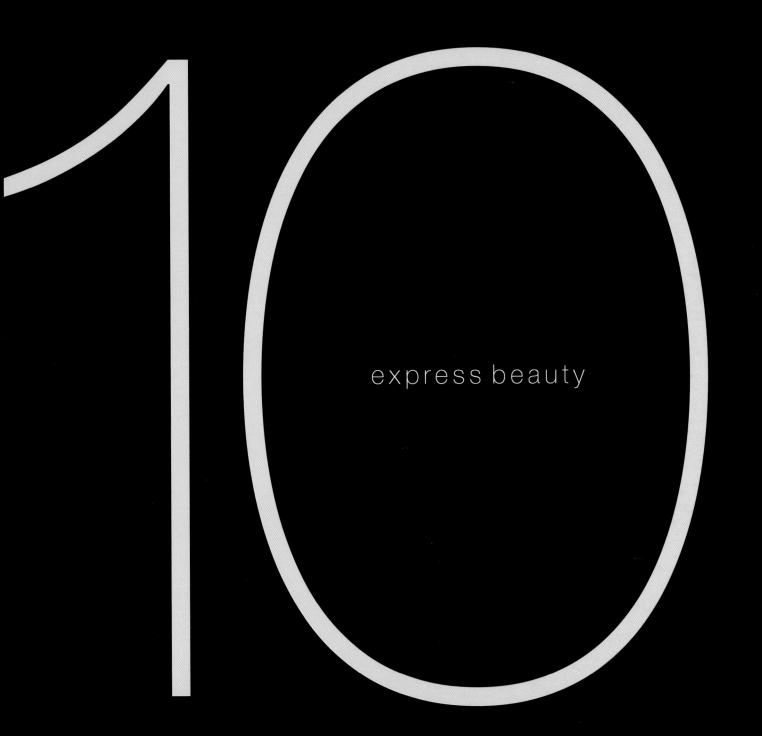

10 express beauty

You can get great results at high speed with quick-fix make-up tips, time-saving hair solutions and short cuts to good grooming. Thankfully, none will compromise your final finish, so when you are pushed for time you can still look your best. This is the ideal way for modern women with hectic lives to devise an appropriate beauty regime.

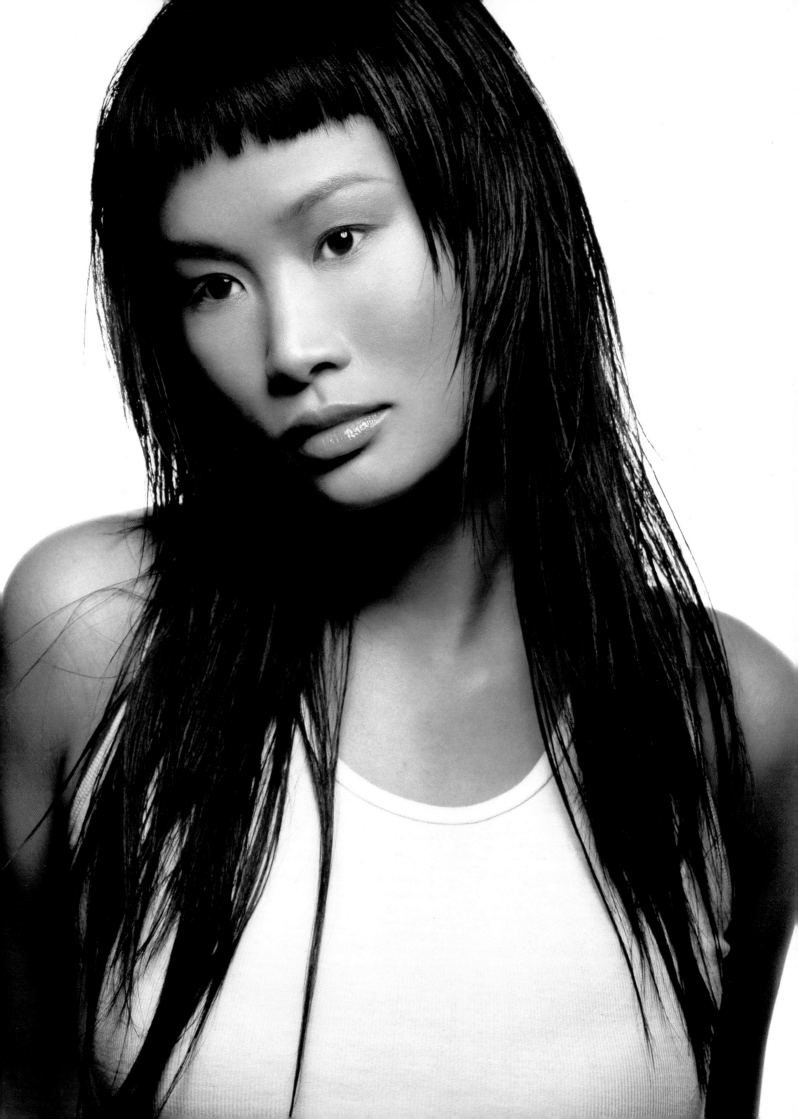

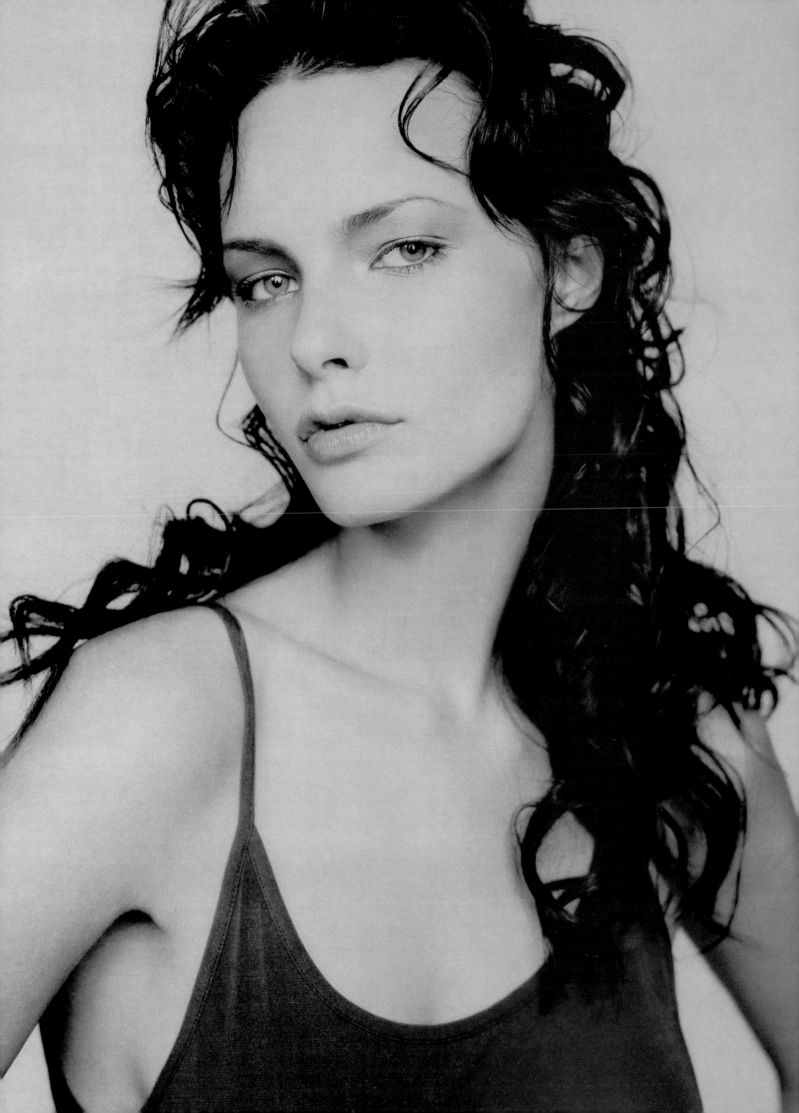

DOUBLE TAKE

Always choose dual-purpose beauty products to save time, or find ways to get more mileage from items you already have in your cosmetic collection when you're racing against the clock.

LIPSTICK Creamy lipsticks in soft shades of pink or rose will double up as blushers. Simply dot them on to the cheek apples and then blend thoroughly into the skin, working in small circular motions, in order to give a natural, healthy-looking finish.

EYESHADOW Let your eyeshadow work as eyeliner too by dampening a fine-tipped make-up brush with water, then dipping it in the eyeshadow and painting it on to add definition.

MASCARA Clear mascara can be used to define the eyelashes and swept through the brows to tame unruly hairs.

PENCIL Invest in a pale-coloured pencil – for example, a soft brown – and use it to add definition to the eyebrows, to outline the eyes and to shade the lips before coating with gloss.

BLUSHER You can get more from a natural shade of cream blusher by using it as lip, eye and cheek colour as well.

BRONZER Use bronzing powder not only to give the face a radiant finish but also to define the eyes, dusting it along the socket line, and to impart a healthy glow to the rest of the body.

MOISTURIZER If you've not had a chance to get to the hairdresser's for a trim, as a temporary solution run an oil-based moisturizer through the ends of the hair to seal split ends.

CONCEALER As well as disguising any blemishes and imperfections, concealer can be used to give lips a hint of colour. Dab it on with the fingertips and then coat with lip balm.

NAIL POLISH If you have snagged your tights and do not have a spare pair with you, you can always paint on a thin film of clear or light-coloured nail polish as an emergency measure to prevent the hole or ladder from getting any bigger.

SHAMPOO Mild shampoos are the perfect travelling companion. As well as handling your hair, they can be used to wash your body and even your clothes. When pushed for time, you should choose a combined shampoo and conditioner.

CONDITIONER Don't splash out on fancy products to use before shaving your legs. Hair conditioner is perfect, with the added advantage of boosting the skin's moisture content.

SERUM During the summer, you can give bare legs a flattering, shiny finish by smoothing hair serum into the skin. Serums that have been enriched with ultraviolet protectors will also help guard the skin against damage from the sun's rays.

GEL If your brows tend to be unruly, a light application of hair gel will slick them into shape and guarantee that they stay put.

WAX If you are wearing leather shoes and suddenly notice that they are scuffed and in need of a shine but you don't have any polish to hand, you can massage hair wax or Vaseline into the leather to add shine, soften it and buff the shoes generally.

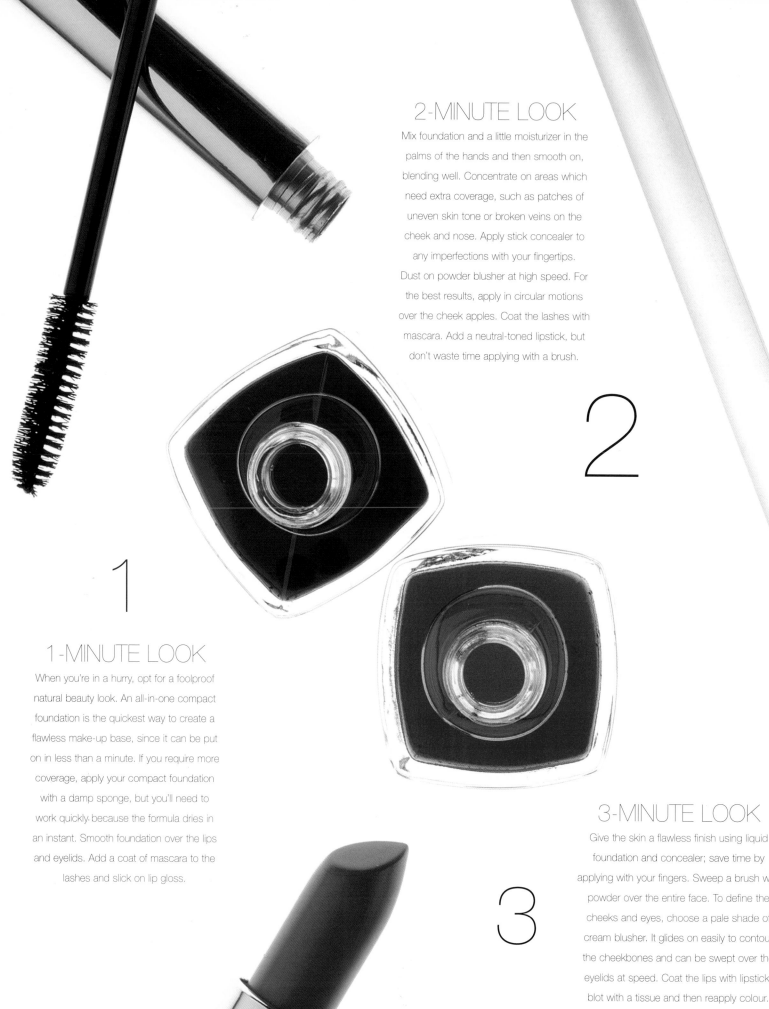

2-MINUTE LOOK

Mix foundation and a little moisturizer in the palms of the hands and then smooth on, blending well. Concentrate on areas which need extra coverage, such as patches of uneven skin tone or broken veins on the cheek and nose. Apply stick concealer to any imperfections with your fingertips. Dust on powder blusher at high speed. For the best results, apply in circular motions over the cheek apples. Coat the lashes with mascara. Add a neutral-toned lipstick, but don't waste time applying with a brush.

1-MINUTE LOOK

When you're in a hurry, opt for a foolproof natural beauty look. An all-in-one compact foundation is the quickest way to create a flawless make-up base, since it can be put on in less than a minute. If you require more coverage, apply your compact foundation with a damp sponge, but you'll need to work quickly because the formula dries in an instant. Smooth foundation over the lips and eyelids. Add a coat of mascara to the lashes and slick on lip gloss.

3-MINUTE LOOK

Give the skin a flawless finish using liquid foundation and concealer; save time by applying with your fingers. Sweep a brush with powder over the entire face. To define the cheeks and eyes, choose a pale shade of cream blusher. It glides on easily to contour the cheekbones and can be swept over the eyelids at speed. Coat the lips with lipstick, blot with a tissue and then reapply colour. Finally, apply your mascara as normal.

six secrets   for fast faces

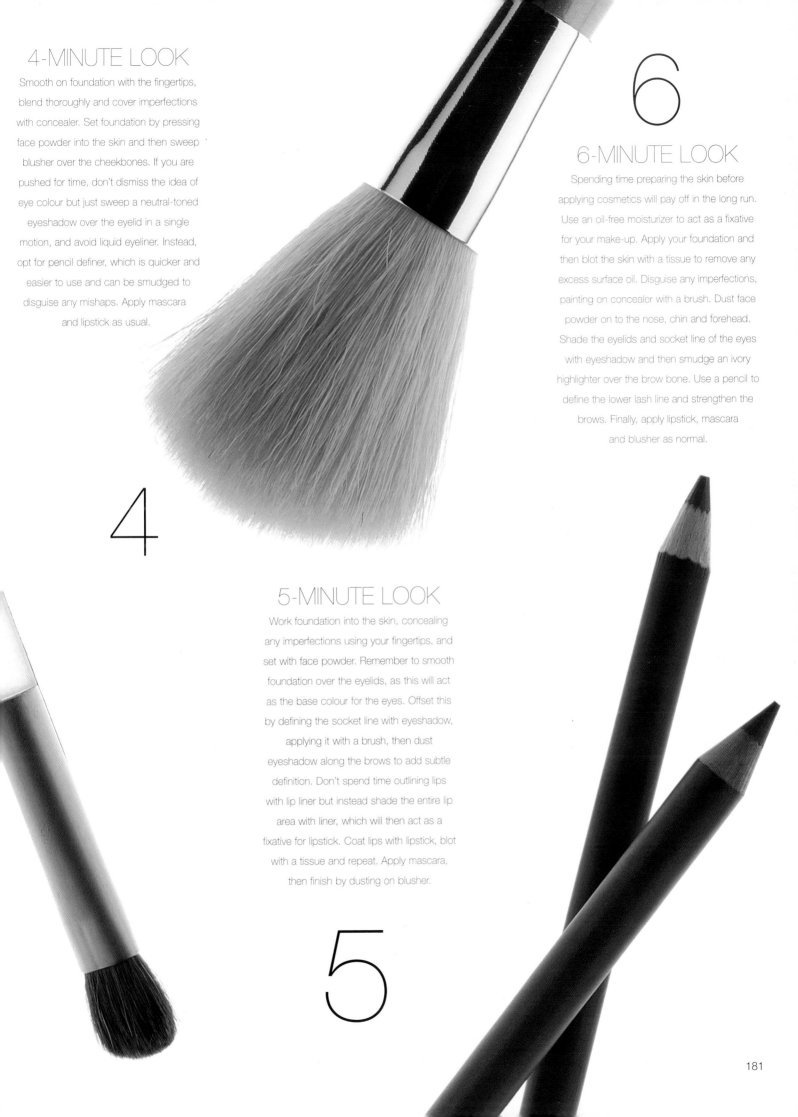

4-MINUTE LOOK

Smooth on foundation with the fingertips, blend thoroughly and cover imperfections with concealer. Set foundation by pressing face powder into the skin and then sweep blusher over the cheekbones. If you are pushed for time, don't dismiss the idea of eye colour but just sweep a neutral-toned eyeshadow over the eyelid in a single motion, and avoid liquid eyeliner. Instead, opt for pencil definer, which is quicker and easier to use and can be smudged to disguise any mishaps. Apply mascara and lipstick as usual.

4

6-MINUTE LOOK

Spending time preparing the skin before applying cosmetics will pay off in the long run. Use an oil-free moisturizer to act as a fixative for your make-up. Apply your foundation and then blot the skin with a tissue to remove any excess surface oil. Disguise any imperfections, painting on concealer with a brush. Dust face powder on to the nose, chin and forehead. Shade the eyelids and socket line of the eyes with eyeshadow and then smudge an ivory highlighter over the brow bone. Use a pencil to define the lower lash line and strengthen the brows. Finally, apply lipstick, mascara and blusher as normal.

5-MINUTE LOOK

Work foundation into the skin, concealing any imperfections using your fingertips, and set with face powder. Remember to smooth foundation over the eyelids, as this will act as the base colour for the eyes. Offset this by defining the socket line with eyeshadow, applying it with a brush, then dust eyeshadow along the brows to add subtle definition. Don't spend time outlining lips with lip liner but instead shade the entire lip area with liner, which will then act as a fixative for lipstick. Coat lips with lipstick, blot with a tissue and repeat. Apply mascara, then finish by dusting on blusher.

5

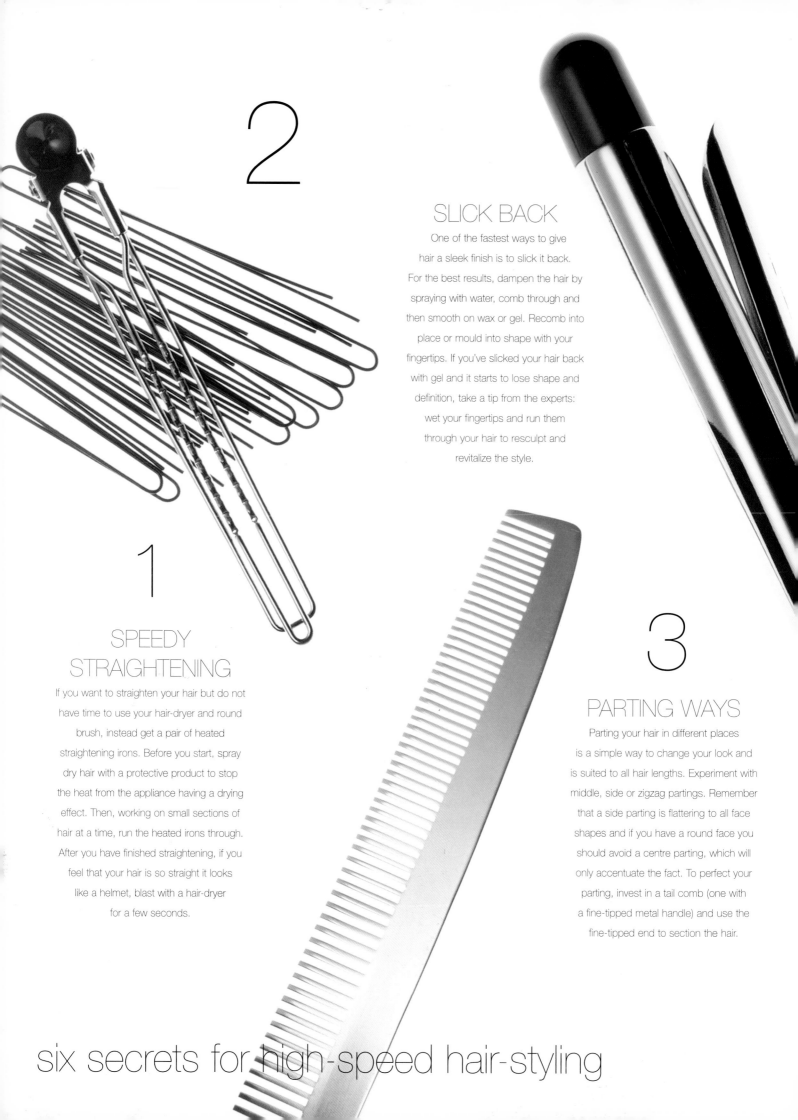

2

SLICK BACK

One of the fastest ways to give hair a sleek finish is to slick it back. For the best results, dampen the hair by spraying with water, comb through and then smooth on wax or gel. Recomb into place or mould into shape with your fingertips. If you've slicked your hair back with gel and it starts to lose shape and definition, take a tip from the experts: wet your fingertips and run them through your hair to resculpt and revitalize the style.

1

SPEEDY STRAIGHTENING

If you want to straighten your hair but do not have time to use your hair-dryer and round brush, instead get a pair of heated straightening irons. Before you start, spray dry hair with a protective product to stop the heat from the appliance having a drying effect. Then, working on small sections of hair at a time, run the heated irons through. After you have finished straightening, if you feel that your hair is so straight it looks like a helmet, blast with a hair-dryer for a few seconds.

3

PARTING WAYS

Parting your hair in different places is a simple way to change your look and is suited to all hair lengths. Experiment with middle, side or zigzag partings. Remember that a side parting is flattering to all face shapes and if you have a round face you should avoid a centre parting, which will only accentuate the fact. To perfect your parting, invest in a tail comb (one with a fine-tipped metal handle) and use the fine-tipped end to section the hair.

six secrets for high-speed hair-styling

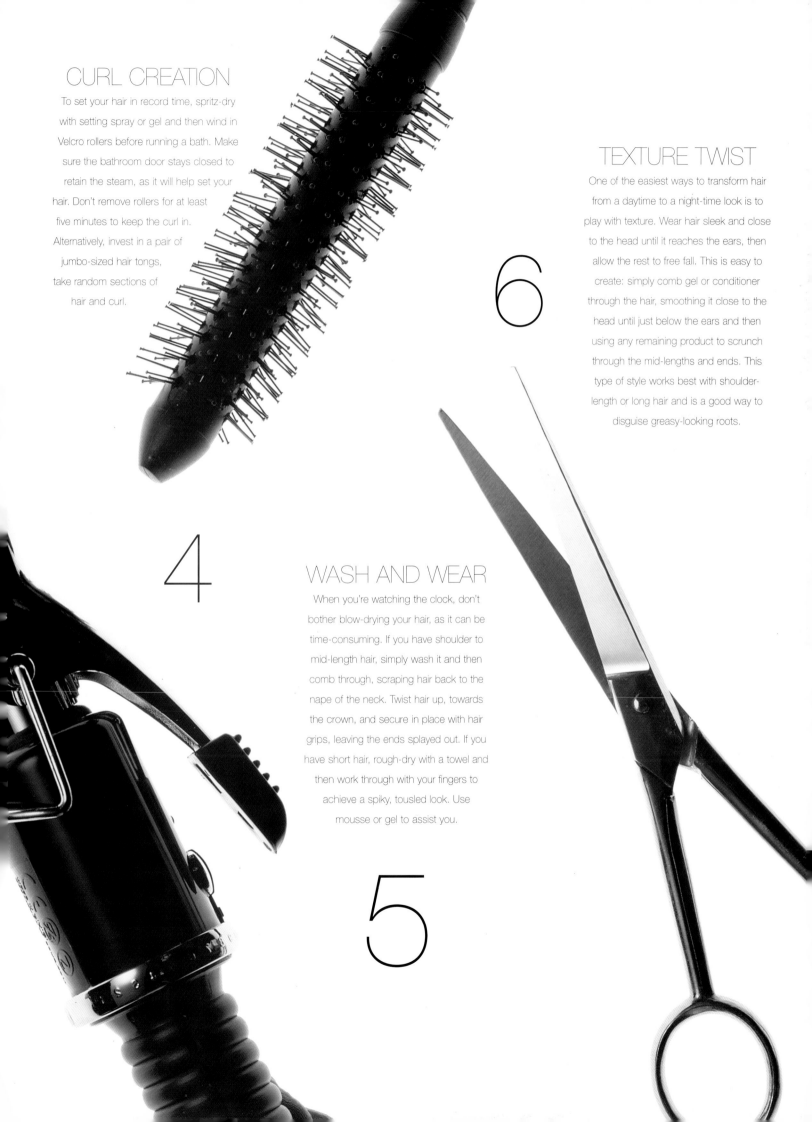

CURL CREATION

To set your hair in record time, spritz-dry with setting spray or gel and then wind in Velcro rollers before running a bath. Make sure the bathroom door stays closed to retain the steam, as it will help set your hair. Don't remove rollers for at least five minutes to keep the curl in. Alternatively, invest in a pair of jumbo-sized hair tongs, take random sections of hair and curl.

TEXTURE TWIST

One of the easiest ways to transform hair from a daytime to a night-time look is to play with texture. Wear hair sleek and close to the head until it reaches the ears, then allow the rest to free fall. This is easy to create: simply comb gel or conditioner through the hair, smoothing it close to the head until just below the ears and then using any remaining product to scrunch through the mid-lengths and ends. This type of style works best with shoulder-length or long hair and is a good way to disguise greasy-looking roots.

6

4

WASH AND WEAR

When you're watching the clock, don't bother blow-drying your hair, as it can be time-consuming. If you have shoulder to mid-length hair, simply wash it and then comb through, scraping hair back to the nape of the neck. Twist hair up, towards the crown, and secure in place with hair grips, leaving the ends splayed out. If you have short hair, rough-dry with a towel and then work through with your fingers to achieve a spiky, tousled look. Use mousse or gel to assist you.

5

INSTANTBEAUTY

PERFECT POUT

Forget all thoughts of surgical implants to plump up your lips. The simplest way to make lips appear fuller is to dab a small amount of gloss on to the centre of the lower lip, either over lipstick or straight on to bare lips. Also, choose pale shades of lipstick to make the lips appear more voluptuous, and avoid dark colours, which will have a slimming effect.

CLEAVAGE ENHANCER

If you are going to wear a plunging neckline, make-up artists recommend that you use a bronze lipstick to enhance your cleavage. Draw a vertical line down the cleavage, then blend into the skin with the fingertips. This will create the illusion that your cleavage is bigger than it really is and will also give the skin a flattering finish.

HAIR VOLUMIZER

If your hair lacks body and volume, add a thickening styling preparation before blow-drying. These usually contain special body-boosting ingredients which are activated by the heat of a hair-dryer. For the best results, tip the head upside-down while blow-drying to ensure that maximum movement is created, then spritz with hairspray to hold.

LUMINOUS SKIN

If your skin needs a tonic, pep up your circulation while applying moisturizer or foundation. For maximum impact, apply with gentle patting motions instead of smoothing on. This will help jump-start blood flow and make the skin look more radiant. Also, put your moisturizer in the fridge for several minutes before applying to give an invigorating boost.

beautifying tips with immediate results

COLOUR RETOUCH

If you have the odd strand of grey hair which you want retouched but don't have time to visit your hairdresser, you can temporarily disguise the problem yourself. Use mascara in the shade closest to your hair colour and coat the strands of grey hair. This will be removed by washing your hair or brushing the colour out.

MOISTURE BOOST

To help disguise wrinkles and fine lines, spray the complexion with a fine mist of water before smoothing on moisturizer. The cells in the skin's upper layers will absorb this water, making them look plumper, and this will make fine lines and wrinkles appear less prominent. Applying moisturizer afterwards will seal this water in, so the effect will last longer.

CUTICLE CARE

If you have unsightly pieces of stray skin around your cuticles, make them look more presentable in an instant by massaging the nail and cuticle with Vaseline. This will also give the nails a high-shine finish. If your fingertips feel greasy afterwards, either wipe with a tissue or use the excess product to tame split ends and give the hair shine.

EYE BENEFIT

Dermatologists are horrified at the thought, but many make-up artists in the film industry will arrive at a shoot armed with a tube of Preparation H. Normally used in the treatment of haemorroids, they swear by it as a quick-fix solution for puffiness around the eyes. Smooth it on and wait: it is the best vasoconstrictor around, although it should only be used occasionally.

BEAUTY INTELLIGENCE

To prevent lip and eye pencils crumbling and breaking when you sharpen them, place them in the fridge for ten minutes first in order to harden the product.

Nail polish can take up to six hours to dry completely, so it is advisable to paint nails before going to bed to avoid doing anything that spoils the finish.

If your eyes are sore and irritated wrap ice cubes in a facecloth and place over closed eyes as a compress. Lie down, chill out and do nothing for five minutes.

To create a French-manicured effect at high speed, try running a white pencil under the nail tips and then painting the nails with a coat of clear or white nail polish.

Wearing peach or apricot blusher will make all faces look youthful, whereas bluish-pink blusher can have an ageing affect, so always take care when choosing colours.

Place a damp make-up sponge in the freezer for a few minutes, then roll over the face to set make-up. It's also a great way to cool down when the heat is on.

6

To make the whites of the eyes appear brighter, use a light blue pencil under the eyes. Soft blue eyeshadow lightly dusted under the eyes will work just as well.

7

When you are applying mascara to the lower lashes, unless you have perfect technique, hold a tissue underneath to prevent mascara collecting on the skin.

8

If you don't have a powder puff or brush with you for applying face powder, a cotton-wool ball dipped in and pressed on to the skin will do the job just as well.

9

One of the quickest ways to transform nasty-looking nails is to add false tips, which can be cut or filed into the size and shape you require in moments.

10

GLOSSARY

ALKALINE
Substances with pH value above 7.

ALPHA HYDROXY ACIDS (AHAs)
Also known as fruit acids, AHAs break down the intercellular glue that binds dead skin cells to the face and body. Using AHA-enriched products buffs away dead skin cells, making skin look more radiant.

ANTIOXIDANTS
Vitamins such as beta carotene, A and E and substances such as green tea and grapeseed extract which counteract the damaging effects of free radicals, which accelerate the ageing process.

CORTEX
Inner layer of the hair shaft which gives hair strength and elasticity. The source of the hair's colour and curl.

CUTICLE
Outer layer of each strand of hair, made up of tiny, overlapping scales. If they don't lie flat, hair will look dull and be more prone to damage.

DERMIS
Second, thicker layer of skin below the epidermis.

EMOLLIENT
Ingredient in skin-care preparations to hydrate and soften the skin.

EPIDERMIS
Thin, outer layer of the skin.

FOLLICLE
Hair follicles in the scalp's dermis are where all the nutrients and oxygen needed for healthy hair growth are found and all growth activity occurs.

FREE RADICALS
Rogue oxidants that are generated by sunlight, pollution, stress and smoking which damage the skin by destabilizing its proper functioning.

HUMECTANT
Ingredient in cosmetic preparations assisting the skin to retain moisture.

HYALURONIC ACID
The skin's natural humectant which attracts water from the air and binds it to the skin. Cosmetic preparations contain it to help hydrate the skin.

HYPOALLERGENIC
Products which have been tested to ensure they won't cause allergic reactions, making them suitable for sensitive, temperamental skins.

KERATIN
Protein found in hair, nails and skin.

MEDULLA
Core or central layer of hair shaft.

MELANIN
Skin and hair's natural pigment.

NON-COMEDEOGENIC
Products formulated to not clog pores, making them ideal for problem, blemish-prone skin.

PH
Scale that determines if a substance is acid or alkaline. Ranging from 0 to 14, 7 is neutral, above 7 is alkaline and below 7 is acid.

PHEOMELANIN
Yellow/red pigments in the cortex that determine natural hair colour.

PORES
Openings of sebaceous glands at skin's surface. Their size is inherited and blocked pores tend to be caused by sebum build-up.

POROUS
Hair which is dry, damaged and has undergone chemical processing is usually porous, meaning that it will quickly and unevenly absorb water or chemicals into the hair shaft.

RELAXED HAIR
Chemical process for straightening Afro hair.

SEBACEOUS GLANDS
Network of tiny glands which are responsible for secreting sebum.

SEBUM
Oily, fatty substance formed in tiny glands round every hair on the body and secreted by the sebaceous glands which acts as lubricant for skin and hair, and helps protect skin.

T-ZONE
Oily area of skin across the forehead, down the nose and chin.

INDEX

DEBBIE PIKE With a degree in graphics and a passion for fashion and beauty, Debbie Pike worked for ten years in London as an art director on magazines such as British *Elle*, *GQ* and *Esquire*. She then moved to Sydney and spent the next two years working on the launch of Australian *marie claire* and for a fashion advertising agency. In 1997 she relocated to New York, where she is now working as a freelance creative director, with many editorial and advertising clients.

DAVID PARFITT The photographs of London-based photographer David Parfitt have appeared in many editorial and advertising projects all over the world during the last fifteen years. Specializing in still-life photography, he is renowned for his innovative approach and ability to make inanimate objects appear exciting and desirable.

TROY WORD Troy Word's desire to be involved in the world of fashion photography took him from Bartlesville, Oklahoma, to the School of Visual Arts in New York City. After graduation and an internship with Albert Watson, he moved to Europe in order to develop his individual style and hone his photographic skills. Today, his work is highly respected worldwide, as indicated by his most recent cosmetic campaigns for Lancôme, Almay and Plenitude by L'Oréal.

Special thanks to Sam Girdwood, Kate Wililams, Sophie Peter, Abigail and Melissa at Shu Uemura, Carrie Kilpatrick, Suzie Cunningham, Emma, Nichole and Claire at Clinique, Sarah Griffith, Natalie Agussol, Daniel at Artomatic, Millie Kendall, Cassandra, Caroline and Susan at Lancôme, Natalie Buckley, Fiona, Owen and Tasia at Dowal Walker PR, Vic Hyde and Rosanna at L'Oréal, Sarah North, Trudi Collister, Grace and Lynette at Whistles, Kathryn Deighton at Muji, Mark Smith at Screen Face and the team at Astrid Sutton Associates, Riverhouse, Karen Berman PR and Felicity Calhrope PR.

Thank you for products and clothing for photography to Clinique, Shu Uemura, Chanel, Christian Dior, Yves Saint Laurent, Estée Lauder, Lancôme, Nars, Stila, Trish McEvoy, Laura Mercier, Issey Miyake, Spectacular, Prescriptives, Gucci, Club Monaco, Paul Mitchell, Bourjois, Iman, The Body Shop, Ruby Hammer, Diamancel, Tweezerman, Boots, No7, Hard Candy, L'Oréal, CP Hart, John Lewis, Original Source, Poppy, Origins, Penhaligons, Czech & Speake, Floris, Toni & Guy, Redken, Aveda, Helena Rubenstein, John Frieda, Charles Worthington, Bulgari, Oribe, L'Occitane, Revlon, BaByliss, Trucco, Vidal Sassoon, Elizabeth Arden, Guerlain, BeneFit, Face Stockholm, MAC, Rimmel, Neal's Yard, Pears, Annick Goutal, La Prairie, L'Clerc, Perfumes Isabell, Jil Sander, Shiseido, Clarins, Philosophy, Jo Malone, Virgin Vie, Crabtree & Evelyn, Bloom, Calvin Klein, Artomatic for their vacuum-packing services, John Smedley, Whistles, Saba, Muji, Aria and Screen Face.

Still-life photos by David Parfitt: back cover, pages 6, 8, 12, 14, 18, 22, 25, 26, 32, 36, 40, 42, 48, 64, 70, 76, 80, 88, 92, 94, 98, 102, 105, 110, 114, 121, 130, 134, 138, 141, 146, 160, 164, 168, 174, 180, 182.

Beauty photos by Troy Word: front cover, pages 11, 17, 21, 35, 39, 51, 52, 55, 56, 59, 60, 61, 62, 63, 73, 74, 79, 83, 91, 97, 101, 113, 117, 118, 122, 125, 133, 137, 149, 150, 152, 153, 154, 155, 163, 167, 177, 178.